Common sense about babies and children

Common sense about babies and children

Dr Hugh Jolly
The Times Paediatrician

Times Newspapers Limited

to the memory of
Moira Keenan

First published in volume form in 1973 by
Times Newspapers Limited, Printing House Square
London EC4P 4DE
Copyright © Times Newspapers Limited 1973
ISBN 0 7230 0094 8

Printed in Great Britain by
Cox and Wyman Ltd.,
London, Reading and Fakenham
Designed by Edward Trott

Contents

INTRODUCTION

Why another book about bringing up children; aren't there enough already? No, considering that this is probably the most important task that any of us undertakes, there are not that many books on the subject. But why do we need a book to tell us how to bring them up anyway – surely it comes naturally? Possibly there was a time when nature did all that was necessary; today, one can see so many unnecessary mistakes being made that I have no doubt of the need for more information being made available. It should even be built into the school curriculum, so that a child will leave school with a real understanding of normal psychology and why people react in the way they do.

Every parent wants to do the best for his children, and this needs a knowledge of child development. The way a baby is treated by his parents, particularly by his mother, determines how he will handle his own children a whole generation later. The 'computer' for this aspect of our behaviour is largely set during the first two or three years of life; if I see a persistently unhappy toddler I can be almost certain that his mother or father had an unhappy childhood.

I must emphasise here that this does not mean you are automatically bound to create problems for your own child if you had an unhappy childhood yourself. Being aware of the possibility will in fact make you more likely to take extra care over the way you handle your child.

I am sometimes asked how permanent an effect the damage done in the early months by bad handling will have on a child. There can be no completely clear answer to this, of course, but I am certain that by understanding what is best for your child at any stage of his life means that you are more likely to provide him with the optimum environment for the full development of his inherent qualities.

1

INTRODUCTION

It is also true to say that anybody who has had a happy childhood is more or less certain to make a happy marriage, and thus to provide a milieu in which his children will thrive. Understanding the importance of this is so much more relevant to a child's well-being than wasting time on worrying about wind or teething troubles.

I wish I knew when the mechanical approach to child care first began. Did they rub babies' backs in Henry VIII's time in order to bring up wind? I doubt it. When did everyone start fussing about the bowels, and what would laxative-makers do if I could persuade parents to stop worrying about their own and their children's bowels!

How can you best tell if your child is thriving and developing normally? First of all, is he energetic? If he is, he will be eating enough. Secondly, does he show a natural curiosity – is he exploring all the time? If so, he has probably got a normal intellect. Normal babies and children have such an inbuilt zest for life that I honestly do not think there is such a thing as a lazy child. If a child seems to be lazy he will in fact be reacting to some way in which his natural development is being mishandled. The area of development in which an anxious parent pressurises his young child will be the one where the child reacts in a negative way, whether this is eating, sleeping, talking or having his bowels open. In the pieces in this book dealing with each of these subjects you will find that again and again I have stressed this important point: when the behaviour of a child goes wrong, you will probably find out why by turning to his parents.

How very different all this is from the old wives' tales that still persist. Some people believe even now that a child needs sleep in order to grow, and that he must have a specific number of hours' sleep each night. In practice, children can often do with less sleep than their parents. How often does one still hear a mother expressing anxiety that her child will not eat anything hot before going off to school in the morning, when there is nothing magical about warm calories and in any case the food put into the stomach soon reaches body temperature, however hot or cold it was when swallowed.

This book includes articles which have appeared in *The Times* during the past three years, as well as containing new material. In editing the articles I have been delighted to find that – such is the speed of progress – some of them contained passages already out of date. A number of paediatricians, as well as general readers, have written to *The Times* asking that these articles should be made available in book form. I am grateful to them for their encouragement and for enabling me to consolidate and expand upon the experiences the articles reflect.

In dedicating this book to Moira Keenan, who was *The Times* Women's Editor, I would like to acknowledge the sympathetic care and skill she brought to her writings on children and their parents and her deep interest in their problems.

PART ONE
FIRST THINGS

1. life before birth

The Chinese have wisely recognised the importance of growth before birth by celebrating the baby's first birthday on the day he is born. Chinese babies are therefore one year older than their counterparts elsewhere.

The baby's weight at birth is determined by two factors: first, the length of time he has been in the womb – a baby born prematurely is naturally smaller than if he had been born at full term; second, the amount of food he has been receiving while in the womb.

Until recently all babies weighing $5\frac{1}{2}$ pounds and under were defined as 'premature'. Only recently has the importance of the underfed baby been appreciated. With it has come a change in terminology, the small baby being called a 'low birth weight baby'. A decision must then be made as to whether this has resulted from a short gestation or a lack of nutrition.

We are often not certain why a baby has been born before the expected date, but the major causes are known to be premature rupture of the membranes and antepartum bleeding from the placenta. The direct cause of a lack of food is an insufficient supply of blood to the developing baby. As the blood contains the baby's food supply, it follows that the more blood the baby receives the greater his size at birth. Twins are sometimes born with widely differing sizes because of an uneven supply of blood from the placenta; the large baby has been receiving much more blood than the smaller one. This difference in size at birth may be so firmly established as to persist throughout life.

The supply of blood to the baby can be reduced by disease of the placenta, as in toxaemia of pregnancy. It is also reduced by smoking. Nicotine is known to diminish the size of arteries, thereby reducing the amount of blood they can carry. It is difficult to imagine any pregnant woman, knowing this, ever considering smoking one more cigarette until her baby has been delivered.

A normal rate of growth while in the womb is a valuable indication that the baby is developing normally. For this reason, the doctor or nurse undertaking an antenatal examination will check the increasing abdominal girth measurement and the rising height of the womb in an attempt to assess the baby's growth. Should the baby's growth cease, the doctor would consider the wisdom of inducing labour since feeding via the placenta is clearly inadequate. Delivery of such a baby could save his life by making it possible for him to be fed by mouth.

It is reasonable to ask how much hereditary factors influence the size of the baby at birth. Interestingly enough, they appear to have very little effect. Their main influence comes after birth, so that the child destined to become a tall adult grows faster immediately after birth, especially during the first six months of life.

By the age of 2 to 3 years any adverse factors leading to a small size at birth are largely removed if optimum nutrition is provided. From that age it therefore becomes possible to predict reasonably accurately the child's ultimate height since he will keep to a standard pattern provided he remains well. Severe illness may cause a temporary slowing up of growth but once recovered from the illness the child grows faster because of 'catch-up growth'. It is believed that there is a central control mechanism in the brain which ensures that the child catches up the lost growth. The body frequently overcompensates so that the child rises above his own curve before coming back on track again. Once back on to his normal track he proceeds along it as though nothing has happened.

aspects of growth 2.

The important point which differentiates a child from an adult is growth. During childhood, every organ in the body is growing, though not all at an equal rate. Each part of the body has its own period in the child's life when it grows fastest, this being known as the 'growth spurt' for that particular organ. The timing of the growth spurt for each organ has a relevance to the function of that organ. Thus the growth spurt for the brain occurs in the last weeks of pregnancy and the first two years of life in human babies. This timing is not the same for each species and no doubt the variation between species relates to the individual needs of that animal. The rat's brain growth spurt occurs mainly after birth whereas this spurt for the guinea pig is considerably before birth. The guinea pig is relatively senile by the time it is born.

The adolescent growth spurt in human children occurs mainly between the ages of 11 and 15 years though, as with every physiological change in the body, there is a small proportion of individuals in whom the change occurs earlier or later than average but in whom it is still perfectly normal.

The age at which the puberty growth spurt occurs can have a profound effect on the child. An early growth spurt leads to early cessation of growth. This means that, after initially becoming taller than the others in his class, the child ends up smaller because the others go on growing for longer and therefore pass him in the end.

Mothers of tall girls who have just had their first period are often very worried lest their daughters will end up as giants, understandably thinking that it heralds the real growth spurt. The knowledge of a straightforward physiological fact may set their minds at rest. The first period occurs on the downward slope of the puberty growth spurt; in other words, the rate of growth is slackening and the child is in fact nearly at the end of her growth period.

There is some evidence to suggest that there is an intellectual advantage in having an early puberty growth spurt. If this is so, such individuals are given an unfair advantage over those with a late growth spurt. It can be used as one more nail in the coffin of the 11+ exam, which by now ought to have been sunk without trace. The only fair system of education is the 'comprehensive', where recognition of a child's potential ability in one area can permit him to be placed with others whose performance is of an equal standard in that subject. Critics of the 'comprehensive' scheme have every reason to complain about the difficulties of fitting it into old-style buildings but they should not try to sink the concept if they are thinking of the child's best interests. And what a great day it will be when handicapped children can be fitted into the appropriate class of the comprehensive school.

Nutrition is of prime importance in the growth of every part of the body. Our belief that Japanese people are small has received a rude shock since the last war because modern Japanese children, with improved nutrition, are considerably taller than their predecessors, though they are not yet as tall as their western counterparts, either because the effects of improved nutrition are incomplete or because there is an inherited element in their smaller stature.

When I was in Japan recently I found I was continually banging my head against the lintel of doors. This was understandable, since I am tall, but what was far more interesting was the number of young Japanese people who were doing the same! Is it possible that pygmies would grow taller if given optimum nutrition and health?

This effect of nutrition on growth has influenced post-war children in the West. However, it does seem likely that we are now nearing an optimum nutrition situation since the ultimate height of the groups most favoured nutritionally seems almost to have reached its peak.

This influence of improved nutrition on growth has also affected the age at the first period. Over the last decades the first period has occurred at a progressively earlier age and the end, as far as this is concerned, is not yet in sight.

In view of this effect of nutrition on growth it is obviously essential to provide optimum conditions for the developing foetus in the womb. The child is growing faster in the womb than at any other time in life including the puberty growth spurt. Measurements after birth show that the rate of growth decelerates rapidly from birth for the first two years of life; it then drops slowly until the puberty growth spurt, which is nothing compared with the speed at which a baby is growing when he comes into the world.

The applications of all this knowledge are enormous. Optimum nutrition must be provided for the baby in the womb, otherwise his brain growth may never pick up. Smoking affects the supply of blood to the body, making the weight of the newborn baby and his brain lighter than average. As a result, he may be permanently less intelligent than he might have been.

Similarly, since the brain growth spurt in human babies occurs in the last weeks of pregnancy and the first two years of life, we must adjust feeding programmes in famine areas. Optimum nutrition must be provided for pregnant mothers and children in the first two years of life in order to ensure maximum growth and development of the brain. Children over the age of two years should be given enough food for survival but, since their brains will not be damaged permanently by starvation, they should not be given a full diet until there is enough food in the area for the needs of all pregnant mothers and small children. It sounds a drastic method of approach to this problem, but it is nevertheless the right way to tackle it.

3. childbirth is a family affair

In our concern for aseptic techniques we must not lose sight of the humanitarian needs of the mother before, during and after the birth of her baby. In the past, childbirth was always a family affair, but despite our increasing emphasis on the need today to support and understand the family, we are allowing it to become less and less so.

It is always safer for labour to take place in hospital rather than at home. This is because delivery requires optimum conditions for the safety of mother and baby. Circumstances can suddenly alter during a normal labour so that the baby's life is placed at risk; everything required for the best method of delivery and for his resuscitation must immediately be at hand. It is for these reasons that doctors recommend delivery in hospital as a routine.

Provided home circumstances are satisfactory and both mother and baby are well, it is ideal that they should return home within forty-eight hours. This not only provides more homely and natural surroundings but also reduces the risk of the baby picking up an infection while in hospital.

Delivery in hospital should not mean a loss of the humanitarian aspects. Progressive obstetric units encourage the father to be present with his wife during delivery in order that they should share this family experience and to enable him to give the support to his wife which only a husband can. This is a demanding role for the husband's emotions for which preparation is needed. Antenatal care should, therefore, include seminars where mothers and fathers are jointly trained in their respective roles during labour.

During the antenatal period those in charge should give advice on the family aspects of the problems as well as on the purely obstetric aspects. Even today some mothers fail adequately to prepare their other children for the new arrival; some believe that a young child, being unable to understand everything, does not need to be told anything. However young the child, he should be given an opportunity to pat his mother's tummy and be told what is going on inside; sometimes he will be lucky enough to feel the baby kicking in the womb. Telling younger children can be left till fairly late on in pregnancy since they do not usually notice the change in a mother's figure and get bored with waiting if told too early.

The father should be advised to keep the children at home with him while his wife is in hospital if he possibly can. Sending the other children away so that they return to find a new baby in the home is bound to increase the chances of jealousy.

All hospitals should encourage visiting of the mother and the new baby by the other children at the earliest opportunity. The risks of introducing infection have been grossly over-exaggerated; this is much more likely to be caused by the doctors, nurses and other hospital staff. The way this first visit is handled is important. The mother should have sufficient warning so that the other children do not find the new baby at her breast, as this will only increase the likelihood of their feeling that their place in the family has been usurped. The baby should be in the cot at the foot of the mother's bed so that the children are likely first to run to their mother's arms to greet her. The mother can then point out the new baby and if she is wise she will have placed an attractively wrapped gift for each child in the cot as a present to them from the new baby. Similarly, it is a happy arrangement if the father has given each child a present to give to their new baby.

In hospital, the place for the baby's cot is alongside his mother's bed – not in the nursery. Babies should only be put in the nursery at night to ensure that the mothers get adequate rest. A mother in a hospital room of her own should be offered the opportunity of having her baby staying with her at night.

By having the baby with her a mother gets to know him much better and she is able to pick him up when he needs her. She will pick him up when he cries, feeding him if necessary, just as she would at home. She will also know that she can bring him into bed with her for play and a cuddle without invoking the wrath of the nurses. There are still some hospitals that disapprove of mothers placing their babies on their beds. This attitude appears to stem from the idea that the counterpane might become infected. Hospitals that keep babies in nurseries produce frightened and ignorant mothers whose problems on returning home are considerably increased.

Early discharge from hospital means an early family reunion in the home. If the mother is staying in the hospital longer than two days she should be encouraged to go out for a meal or a walk with her husband. It should be explained that the hospital staff will act as babysitters for nothing. This helps the father to adjust to the new relationship with his wife, unhindered by the presence of his baby. It also ensures that the mother has faced up to the first occasion when she leaves her new baby in someone else's care and when she goes out into the world again.

The interests of the family are best served by a humanitarian and non-rigid attitude from the hospital staff; family problems will be lessened and the chances of maternal depression reduced.

getting to know the new baby 4.

Probably the first thing you will want to know as soon as your baby is born is whether it is a boy or a girl. After that you will want to know if he's normal – if everything is there and in its right place. Provided the doctor or midwife who has taken charge of the delivery is understanding and sympathetic the baby will be put in your arms as soon as they have checked that he is breathing safely. This is far more important than bathing or weighing. A maternity sister once said to me that she felt the labour had gone perfectly only if she got the baby to the breast before the delivery of the afterbirth.

The ritual of bathing the newborn baby has changed considerably. After his exhausting journey down the birth canal the baby has earned a rest instead of being plunged immediately into a bath. Moreover, the baby gets cold very easily in the first few minutes after he has left the warmth of his mother and bathing may exaggerate this so that his temperature falls considerably. At birth, the skin is covered by a greasy substance called vernix; this has been produced by the same glands that are responsible for the greasiness of normal skin. The vernix stays for a few days if it is not removed by bathing and there is some evidence that it acts as a protection against infection. This is another reason why some doctors are against the early bath, being satisfied with 'topping and tailing' at this stage so that the face, head and bottom only are cleaned.

When you slide your hand over the top of the baby's head you will find a shallow area called the soft spot or anterior fontanelle. The bones making up the skull are not united at birth in order to allow for growth of the head. The contour of these bones creates a diamond-shaped gap on the top of the head which gradually closes during the first twelve months of life. This gap in the bones is covered by a thick membrane providing a very safe protection for the underlying brain. Mothers should therefore have no fear of washing the baby's head, including the soft spot, although the presence of scurf over the spot is a common sign that a mother has been frightened to wash there. On one occasion a mother found the soft spot for the first time when her baby was 10 days old; she came to me in a terrible state saying, 'Doctor, I've broken his head.' I felt that her anxieties resulted from insufficient time being spent with her by the doctors and nurses in the early days when they should explain as much as possible about the newborn baby and answer her questions.

All babies are checked by the doctor or midwife immediately after birth to make sure there is no major problem present. Within the next twenty-four hours the doctor should carry out a detailed examination, as he would for any other new patient coming under his care. Ideally, this examination should be undertaken with the mother present – her bed makes a good examination couch – so that she can see what he is doing and ask any questions she wants. One of the tests the doctor will make is to check that the hips are not dislocated and that there is no tendency to dislocate. It is by this means that the consequences of congenital dislocation of the hip, which used to be a fairly common cause of serious disability, can be eradicated by early treatment.

The umbilical cord will already have been tied and should be left alone unless there is any sign of oozing of blood. Bleeding from the cord is very rare now that it is tied with an elastic band or a special clamp is used. Both of these maintain continuous pressure as the cord shrinks during the early hours of life, and are much more effective than the old type of cotton thread used which sometimes worked loose.

Mixed with excitement at the arrival of the new baby a mother may feel fear and even panic lest she fails to look after him properly. Being aware that she now has a helpless baby, utterly dependent on her, may make her wonder if she will ever feel safe again since she is now infinitely vulnerable. It is these feelings and the changes, both chemical and physical, going on inside her, which account for many mothers feeling miserable and bursting into tears, especially when the baby is about three days old.

Another reason for a mother's misery and bewilderment in these early days is the mistaken belief that the mother automatically loves her new baby totally. This is far from true – it takes time to fall in love with anyone, including your own newborn baby.

the risks of inherited disorders 5.

A major thought of every expectant mother is: 'Will my baby be normal?' Closely tied up with this fear is the possibility of some inherited abnormality. This will be considered even more seriously by the parents if the baby is born malformed, or if later events show the baby to have a congenital disorder of the type which is not apparent at birth.

Our knowledge of inherited disorders is increasing all the time, though much still remains to be understood. 'Genetic counselling', whereby parents are told of the possible risks for their future children, is now an established part of the advice available. It may be given by the family doctor or by a hospital consultant, particularly a paediatrician or an obstetrician. Alternatively, the more specialised advice of a geneticist may be required. Specialists in genetic disorders are mainly hospital based, and those needing advice would be referred to the genetic clinic by the family doctor or by one of the hospital consultants.

The risk of the inheritance of certain disorders is clear-cut, the two major varieties being dominant and recessive. Dominant inheritance – the less common of the two – requires that one parent already suffers from the disorder. In consequence, half the children will be similarly affected. An example of this method of inheritance is achondroplasia – the disorder which often accounts for those dwarfs seen performing in a circus.

Recessive inheritance requires that both parents should be carriers of the same disease. They will not have the disease themselves but one in four of their children will be affected. Two out of four of their children will be healthy carriers like themselves, and one out of four will be totally unaffected. It is probable that everyone carries recessive genes capable of producing disease in their offspring, but this occurs only if the other parent also carries the same recessive gene. An example of a recessively inherited disease is cystic fibrosis. This does not usually show itself at birth, but at an early age the smell of the child's stools becomes very offensive because of imperfect digestion and he is likely to develop repeated chest infections.

The risk of a recessively inherited disorder could be put another way by saying that three out of every four children will be normal, although two of these will be carriers. The risk in each pregnancy remains the same whatever the result of the previous pregnancy. If a coin is tossed in the air and turns up heads on three successive occasions, the chance for heads or tails on the next toss remains unaltered.

So far, inheritance seems to be a fairly clear-cut process, but unfortunately genes do not always run true to type. They are liable to undergo a change, called a mutation, which completely alters the odds and is one reason why the advice of a geneticist is sought. The task of the family doctor or the specialist whom he consults is to decide whether the disorder suffered by the child is of the inherited type. In this case genetic advice may be given by the first doctor or he may refer the parents for more specialised advice.

Some recessive genes are linked to the X sex chromosome so that only boys are affected by the disease although it is the girls who are the carriers. Haemophilia is an example of such a disorder. It was carried by Queen Victoria and passed by her to a number of her male descendants.

In giving genetic advice the doctor will not tell the parents what to do about having or not having any more children. This is a decision which they must make for themselves once they have been given all the information available and in a form in which they can understand it.

Certain forms of mental handicap are inherited, and it is the doctor's responsibility with every backward child to tell the parents whether or not their child has an inherited form of backwardness. The majority of backward children do not have an inherited disease.

Mongolism is one variety of backwardness which may be inherited. The majority of mongols do not result from inherited disorders; it is usually due to the older age of the mother. This is due to a failure of the fertilised ovum to divide itself equally in the earliest stage of development of the baby. Increasing age seems to make the ovum less efficient at normal division. The very small proportion of mongols resulting from an inherited disorder can be determined by a blood test carried out on the mongol baby. Because of the increased risk of mongolism in older mothers it is now possible to test the amniotic fluid which surrounds the baby in the womb to decide if the baby in the womb is a mongol. This is a very complicated test which involves growing, in a tube, some of the skin cells shed by the baby. It is not yet a routine test but it is an example of one further way in which the science of genetic counselling is advancing.

6. babies born malformed

There can be few expectant mothers who have not worried lest their baby will be born deformed. So often, therefore, the first question a mother asks her doctor or midwife is whether her baby is normal, as well as settling down herself to check the baby all over.

Public awareness of the problem has been increased by the thalidomide disaster, which has had one advantage in that it has stimulated more research into the causes of congenital malformations. Not so very long ago it would have seemed absurd to talk of preventing such deformities but now everyone knows that some can be prevented.

The size of the problem is vast; approximately one in every fifty babies born has a severe malformation. There are also an unknown number of miscarriages due to this cause. However, considering the complexity of human development it is not surprising that errors occur; in fact, it is remarkable that they do not occur more often.

A major stimulus to research into the causes of

these malformations has been the reduction in infant mortality from other causes, following improvement in the overall care both of mothers and of babies. A high infant mortality rate means an emphasis on other preventable problems, particularly infection. In western countries we are now reaching the hard core of causes of infant mortality so the importance of congenital malformations looms larger.

Any influence causing an abnormality in the baby must act before the twelfth week of foetal life, since by that age all the organs of the foetus are fully formed. After this age growth of the organs can be affected adversely, for example by smoking, but not their development.

Knowledge of which malformations are inherited and which are not is essential for doctors in order for them to advise parents of possible risks in future pregnancies.

A number of viruses causing infection in the mother can be transmitted to the baby in her womb. Of these, German measles is the most important. It can cause deafness and blindness as as well as damage to the developing brain and heart. Vaccination against German measles is now available for girls aged from 11 to 14 years. Mothers of these young girls should make sure that their daughters' future babies are protected by this major advance in medicine.

Thalidomide highlighted the risk of damage from drugs, and it is likely that many medicines can cause damage. Such medicines are particularly prescribed for sickness in the early months but the only safe advice is to avoid them altogether. X-rays can have a damaging effect, so the mother's routine chest X-ray is left until after the third month of pregnancy.

Mechanical factors operating inside the uterus can also cause malformations of the baby. The baby can be literally squashed over a period of weeks so that one or more limbs are deformed. This is the most common cause of club feet and is also one factor in congenital dislocation of the hip. The normal newborn baby adopts the position in which he has been lying in utero for the past weeks. For this reason he is usually bent up in a flexed position. In view of the strength of the forces involved it is not surprising that compression does sometimes cause the body to be malformed.

A surprising but major factor in the production of congenital malformations is the mother's socio-economic state. The poorer this is, the greater the likelihood of malformations. In the British Perinatal Survey of 1958, mothers from social class 5 (husbands – unskilled workers) had six times the number of malformed babies as did mothers from social class 1 (husbands – professional workers). This is but one more piece of evidence to emphasise how dependent the health of a nation is on improved socio-economic conditions.

7. about rhesus disease

The major blood factors are A, B and O so that in any blood transfusion careful matching of these factors between the blood of the donor and the blood of the patient is essential. Many other factors are carried in the blood and from the point of view of the unborn baby it is the rhesus factor which is the most important.

The name rhesus was given to this factor because it was shared with the rhesus monkeys. 85 per cent of white men and women are 'rhesus positive', indicating that they carry this factor. 15 per cent are therefore rhesus negative and it is rhesus negative women who are at risk. For negro people, the chance of being rhesus negative is only about 1 per cent so that this problem is much less common in negroes.

Rhesus disease only affects the baby and this can occur if a rhesus positive man marries a rhesus negative woman and gives her a rhesus positive baby. The baby's and the mother's blood circulation pass very close to each other in the placenta (afterbirth). In fact, at one point only one layer of cells separates the two bloods. During labour, when the placenta is squeezed, some red blood cells from the baby commonly escape into the mother's circulation. This does not harm the mother; problems only arise if the baby is rhesus positive and the mother rhesus negative. In this case the baby's red cells stimulate the mother to form rhesus antibodies which circulate in her blood. These antibodies are capable of passing across the placenta into the baby's circulation.

The same situation can occur if a rhesus negative mother is given a blood transfusion of rhesus positive blood. It is to be hoped that this would never happen today.

Since antibody production takes some weeks, the baby who causes the problem is not affected by rhesus disease, having left the womb while all was still well. Thus first-born babies of rhesus negative mothers are seldom affected; it is the next rhesus positive baby conceived by this rhesus negative mother who is likely to be affected.

In the case of the second rhesus positive baby, antibodies from the mother pass across into the baby's circulation while he is still in the womb. These antibodies destroy many of the baby's red cells so that the baby may die while still in the womb or may be born anaemic and rapidly develop severe jaundice. Such babies have to have their blood changed at or soon after birth in order to get rid of as much of the rhesus antibody infected blood as possible. This exchange blood transfusion may need to be repeated once or more often during the early days of life.

Tests while the baby is still in the womb can discover whether he is being affected by rhesus disease. If the baby is being severely affected it is possible to give him a blood transfusion while still in the womb, by injecting the blood into the baby's abdomen. This injection of blood avoids the intestines, and the blood is absorbed into his circulation.

Severely affected babies, whether or not they have needed a blood transfusion while still in the womb, are likely to have labour induced early in order to reduce the severity of the disease. They must be delivered in a hospital where full facilities for an immediate exchange transfusion are available.

So far, I have explained the reasons for rhesus disease in babies and how it is treated. However, modern research has now gone a long way to preventing the disease. The baby's rhesus positive red cells which escaped into the mother's circulation during labour can be destroyed by giving the mother an injection of rhesus antibody. They will not therefore survive long enough to stimulate permanent antibody production by the mother. The rhesus antibody used for the injection has come mainly from male volunteers. Since it is injected into the mother it only lasts a few weeks and therefore raises no problems for the next baby.

It is now a routine to test the blood of rhesus negative mothers as soon as the baby and the placenta have been delivered. In this way it is possible to discover whether any of the baby's red cells have got into the mother's circulation. If they have, the mother is given an injection of antibodies so as to destroy these red cells before they can cause any permanent problem by stimulating her system to form antibodies.

Women who developed rhesus antibodies in their blood because of pregnancies before this advance in treatment cannot have these antibodies removed. For them it will be a matter of treating their subsequent babies if these are affected.

In the future, there is every hope that the rhesus problem for babies will be wiped out, provided these very careful checks are kept on the mother and the correct treatment given.

breast-feeding or . . . 8.

Shall I breast-feed my baby? This is the question to be faced by all mothers, and it should be discussed during pregnancy. A surprising number of babies are born whose mothers have apparently not considered the question beforehand.

Mothers are often put off the idea of breast-feeding by the prejudiced and ignorant remarks of relatives and friends, so it is important to get a few facts clear. What are the advantages of breast-feeding? In this country, where the risk of infection (gastroenteritis) from dirty bottles and teats is low, the main reason for recommending breast-feeding is the close emotional tie it helps to create between mother and baby. This does not mean that such a tie is impossible without breast-feeding, but it is encouraged by a mother feeding her own baby. It is a unique experience to watch a baby grow and to realise that this has all come from the mother without the aid of any other source of food for the baby; the thrill this gives to mothers is not surprising.

Preparation for breast-feeding begins during the antenatal period, when the doctor or midwife should discuss the pros and cons of the subject, giving the mother the opportunity to express her own feelings and doubts and helping her to resolve these. The breasts will be examined and sometimes treatment is required for flat nipples so that by the time the baby is born these have been drawn out. Old-fashioned methods to harden the nipples are quite incorrect; nothing special needs to be done for the normal nipple.

When the baby is born he is cuddled at the breast as soon as possible – ideally before the after-birth is delivered. This is not to give him a feed, since the breast does not fill up with milk until about two days after birth, but to help the mother get to know her baby better at an early stage.

During the first two days the baby is put to the breast for comfort and cosiness rather than for a feed. A few babies are thirsty during this time and can be given boiled water to drink but most are happy to rest, with an occasional cuddle, until the milk arrives.

Once the breasts fill up with milk its actual flow is largely conditioned by the baby. Holding the baby in her arms will stimulate the flow of milk which is still further encouraged by the baby sucking. Suction on the nipple causes messages to be sent to the pituitary gland in the brain which then releases a chemical messenger (oxytocin) which causes the strands of muscle surrounding the breast cells to contract. This produces a flow of milk from the breast, usually in drops but sometimes in a jet. The message is sent to both breasts so that a flow of milk also comes from the breast not being sucked by the baby. This flow from the other breast occurs mainly at the beginning of each feed and tends to lessen as the early weeks are passed.

Any sudden noise or embarrassment may counteract the messages from the brain so that the flow of milk ceases. This reaction varies with different mothers according to their temperament, accounting for their differing ability to feed or not when other people are about.

In the early days a mother may feel that breast-feeding is messy and she may not like the smell of milk around her. Such feelings usually sort themselves out rapidly so that they soon recede into the background.

During the feed a mother may experience colicky pains in the lower part of her abdomen. These are an exaggeration of the normal after-pains caused by the contractions of the womb as it goes back to its former size. This contraction is brought about by the same messenger (oxytocin) as causes the flow of milk and is nature's way of ensuring a rapid reduction in size of the womb; this is one of the advantages of breast-feeding.

There is no need to drink enormous amounts of water while breast-feeding. Mothers need only drink the amount they feel they need; an excess causes nausea and unnecessarily frequent visits to the lavatory.

The breast works similarly to the widow's cruse: the more milk that is taken off the greater its supply. This is an important difference from the ordinary jug of water and must be explained to mothers who otherwise, when supplies are short, are liable to try storing up milk for the evening feed. In fact, this has the reverse effect and reduces the supply, whereas frequent feeds increase the supply.

Once breast-feeding has been established it is simpler to manage than bottle-feeding. Many a husband has blessed its convenience during the night when otherwise he might have been sent downstairs to prepare a bottle.

Some husbands fear the loss of their wife's figure as a result of breast-feeding but this is unlikely if a good bra is worn. The alteration in breast shape after the first baby is probably due to physiological changes resulting from having a baby rather than from actually feeding him.

A greater understanding of breast-feeding increases the number of parents wishing their babies to be fed this way. At the same time, doctors and midwives must not be so enthusiastic about breast-feeding that they leave those mothers who are unable or unwilling to breast-feed feeling that they have failed their baby.

bottle-feeding 9.

When I was a medical student, the subject of artificial feeding was taught as such a complicated subject that I found it hard to believe I would ever master it. However, when I qualified and started working with babies I realised that it was really a very simple subject, requiring knowledge of a few basic facts but not the mass of scientific detail I had been made to learn.

I believe that many mothers approach the subject with similar trepidation. The very term

'formula' adopted by the Americans to describe
a baby's milk mixture suggests a need for
scientific precision. Whereas, provided a baby is
healthy, I am certain that this sort of accuracy of
detail is unnecessary.

Why then were the pioneers of child care in the
first half of this century so adamant about the
need for accuracy? These teachers would hand
out long tables of instructions giving details of
the quantity and strength of each feed as the baby
grew, together with the exact interval which was
to be allowed between each feed.

I suspect that this was a reflection of the much
more mechanical approach to child-rearing then
in vogue. The baby seems to have been regarded
as a machine which had to be fed to order and
regularly checked to see that it emptied itself
properly. It was not unusual in children's hospitals
for the consultant to check the previous day's
stools which were laid before him and then to
pronounce on what changes in the baby's feeds
were required. Even today I meet many mothers
who spend all their time thinking about their
baby's feeds and the appearance of his stools.

Of course, the earlier paediatricians had to
contend with serious outbreaks of infectious
diarrhoea which must have influenced their approach to the subject of feeding. Standard
methods of sterilisation of feeds were still only
being considered.

In what ways, therefore, can we now simplify
the approach to bottle-feeding? First by em-
phasising that all the manufactured milks are
equally good and that babies can be fed just as
well on dried milk or evaporated (condensed)
milk, keeping to the simple instructions printed
on the packet or the can. There is never any need
to change the milk on the grounds that the first
one did not suit the baby. A healthy baby can
take any of them equally well.

The type of milk is sometimes changed because
a baby is being sick, but most often this sickness is
nothing more than simple regurgitation which is

very common and does the baby no harm. If the baby is really vomiting up his feeds a doctor's advice is needed.

Going off feeds is never a reason for changing the milk. A baby who suddenly stops feeding needs a doctor at once because this is the classic way in which an infection shows itself in babies.

Ordinary table sugar (sucrose) is just as good as any other form of sugar. There is no need to spend extra money by making up the milk feeds with glucose since sucrose is converted to glucose in the baby's stomach. Neither is there any advantage in brown sugar over white.

A great deal of unnecessary time is wasted in getting the milk to the 'correct' temperature. Provided the milk is not too hot it does not matter what the temperature is. Whenever I get the chance I give a baby a bottle of milk straight out of a refrigerator – I am still looking for a baby who refuses it! Most adults prefer cold milk to hot milk, so why should not the baby?

It is the mother's feelings which determine the the time she spends on getting the milk to the 'correct' temperature. Understandably, she is likely to think the milk should be at body temperature, the same as breast milk, but the baby is much more liberal in his outlook.

A common error with bottle-feeding is to be concerned if the baby does not finish all the milk. But provided he has started off normally, the amount he takes at any one feed does not matter. Breast-fed babies vary enormously in the amount they take at different feeds but no one worries about this because it is not obvious. If bottles were opaque and were thrown away when the baby had finished the problem would be less.

The time interval between feeds should be determined by the baby. 'Demand' feeding is now almost universal for breast-fed babies, but because cow's milk feeding is 'artificial' there is a greater tendency to keep to an artificial interval, determined by the clock.

Provided the bottle is held at a slope so that the

teat is filled with milk, there is no need to worry
about wind. Repeatedly stopping the feed to bring
up the baby's wind is unnecessary and often
makes him cry because the feed has been taken
away from him. A baby will always burp if he
needs to – he can't stop himself.

The big thing about artificial feeding is to give
the bottle lovingly. It cannot feel and smell like his
mother's breast but if a baby is cradled closely in
his mother's arms while being bottle-fed he is
much more cosy than if he is held facing his
mother and is fed like a bird.

10. attitudes to circumcision

The other day a mother asked me why it was so
difficult to get baby boys circumcised these days.
She was not referring to ritual or tribal circumcision but only to those operations undertaken
for medical reasons. The answer to this question is
straightforward – doctors are not in favour of unnecessary operations and they are now aware that,
in the past, circumcision was frequently carried
out for no good medical reason.

Twenty years ago a doctor undertook an important piece of research showing that at birth
the foreskin and the end of the penis are united.
In the womb, the whole of the penis, including the
foreskin, develops from a single bud. Separation
of foreskin from penis occurs slowly during the
early years of life, being completed some time
between the first and third year. It will be obvious,
therefore, that the term 'phimosis', meaning a
tight foreskin, should never be applied at birth
and on no account should a doctor, nurse or
mother push back the foreskin of a newborn
baby. If this is done, the union between foreskin
and penis is torn, as the frequent bleeding caused
by this manoeuvre shows. The tear heals by scarring, as with any other body tear. In this case it
causes the foreskin to adhere permanently to the
penis so that it now cannot be pulled back. This

is 'phimosis' which, it will now be appreciated, is man-made and may require circumcision for correction.

The correct advice for the mother of a newborn baby boy is to leave the foreskin strictly alone so that natural separation is not interfered with. When her boy is about three or four years old she will find that it is easy to push back the foreskin; for the first few occasions this is most easily carried out in the bath.

With this swing away from circumcision, doctors are now asked about the disadvantages of the operation. The major one is that it is wrong to subject a baby to an unnecessary operation and one which carries risks, even though these are very few. Twenty years ago the doctor who undertook the research already described found that in this country there was then a yearly toll of some sixteen child deaths from the operation. A less dramatic disadvantage results from removal of the protective covering which the foreskin provides for the end of the penis. During infancy, the penis is often soaked in a wet napkin; if circumcised, its end is very liable to become inflamed leading to an ulcer at the end of its opening. This 'meatal' ulcer heals by scarring and is therefore liable to cause narrowing of the opening.

The increased risk of cancer of the neck of the womb in women married to uncircumcised men is related to inadequate male hygiene. It can be entirely prevented by normal hygienic measures to keep the foreskin clean.

Circumcision started as a religious ritual, but with the rise of modern surgery in the last century its status changed from a religious rite to that of a common surgical operation. It also has a connection with differences in social class, being more commonly found among boys at public schools than those at state schools, an association that has also applied to the removal of tonsils and adenoids in the past. It is interesting that with both these operations parents assume the role of

doctor and are prepared to decide that the
operation is necessary, something they would
never do with a hidden organ such as the appendix.

PART TWO
ATTITUDES TO ILLNESS

11. when to call the doctor

The short answer is: whenever you are worried and feel you need his help. You are the only person who knows whether you are so worried that you need the advice of a doctor. But that doesn't mean you have to call him out – you may easily be able to get the advice and reassurance you need by making a telephone call. More and more doctors are encouraging mothers to seek this advice by telephone, since it saves time for both parties. At least one family doctor has installed a telephone in his car, as he finds that if he settles the anxieties of his patients as soon as they arise there is still further saving of time, since the anxieties, being less deeply ingrained, can be dealt with more easily. In America many paediatricians have two separate 'telephone hours' during the day, commonly from 8 a.m. to 9 a.m. and 5 p.m. to 6 p.m., when parents can ring in for a telephone consultation.

If the telephone is unavailable or unsuitable for the consultation a mother should do her best to bring her child round to the surgery rather than calling the doctor out to her home. Modern family doctors (general practititioners) run an appointment system so that she will see the doctor with the minimum of waiting. Obviously, if she suspects her child has an infectious illness the child must not be brought into a waiting room where he could infect other children, but many more children could be brought to the surgery instead of calling out the doctor. A child with a fever is unlikely to come to any harm by being taken to the doctor in a car or pram, and if he is severely ill he will in any case have to be taken out of doors in order to travel to the hospital.

The basic question behind the majority of fears felt by a mother during the early years of her child's life is whether her child is healthy, even though the question she asks relates to eating, sleeping or bowels. The best sign of health is energy, and as long as a child maintains his normal activity the actual amount of food he eats does not matter. Cars differ in the number of miles they do to a gallon of petrol; in the same way children vary in the amount of energy they extract from a given quantity of food. This difference relates to the individual's capacity to change his food into energy.

The importance of appetite as an assessment of a child's health is when it is suddenly lost. This is a sure sign that something is wrong, usually indicating an infection, particularly in young babies. Of all the danger signals which mothers need to be taught about their babies, this is the most important.

This is something which particularly needs to be taught to mothers in developing countries, where infection is very common but the early signs of ill health not understood. I was recently teaching the medical students in the Ghana Medical School when the mother of a six-month-old baby arrived complaining in local language that he had a worm in his belly – a common complaint. After examining her baby I was delighted to be able to tell her that her child was entirely healthy. The next mother to come in had a similar complaint about her baby but this one was dead in her arms. She had failed to appreciate the seriousness of his loss of appetite which he had had for some time.

A rise in temperature is a poor guide to the health of a baby. Some babies may be perfectly well despite a rise in temperature above the so-called normal figure of 98·4°F (37°C), whereas a baby may be very ill when the temperature is below this figure. A low temperature sometimes accompanies a severe infection in a baby because it has knocked out his heat regulating mechanism. It is for this reason that doctors and nurses use a low-reading thermometer when taking a baby's temperature, since it goes down to 85°F (29·4°C) instead of 95°F (35°C) as on the ordinary thermometer. For this reason, when a mother telephones her doctor to say her child is ill the doctor should first inquire whether he is taking his feeds normally rather than whether he has a fever. Sadly, some mothers have been made to feel they cannot telephone their doctor when worried about their child unless the child has a temperature.

Vomiting is another serious symptom. A single vomit may not be serious but if it persists, particularly in a child who is seldom sick, the child must be seen by a doctor.

Diarrhoea is a common symptom in children, not only resulting from an infection in the bowels themselves but commonly accompanying infections anywhere in the body, for example in the throat or ears. It may also result from something unsuitable having been eaten. In most cases diarrhoea alone is not an emergency, but if it persists, and particularly if it is associated with vomiting, a doctor should see the child.

Constipation seldom requires an urgent call to a doctor. Most often a mother's concern about her child's bowels relates to her own mistaken belief that bowels must be open every day lest the 'poisons' in the bowels are absorbed into the system. Constipation associated with vomiting and with distension of the stomach is always serious, being due usually to obstruction of the intestines; fortunately this is rare. A change in bowel habit should be noted and may be something to mention to the doctor but not as an emergency unless the child is obviously ill.

A mother must feel free to contact her doctor whenever she is worried because she is the best judge of the situation. She should always call him if she feels her child is ill, particularly, let me emphasise again, if he has gone off his food. No good doctor will scold a mother for calling him on the telephone when she is worried.

12. first aid

Parents should know enough first aid to be able to deal with the common accidents which befall their

children, particularly cuts and burns. The subject
is not as complicated as many people think. The
first need is to have the requisite equipment. This
equipment should be kept together in a special
box, clearly marked 'first aid'. It should always
be left in the same place in the house so that
everyone knows where to find it in an emergency.
A good place to keep the box is in the kitchen
since this is the most common room in the house
for accidents to occur. In addition, the kitchen is
often the most convenient and accessible room
for treating children returning home after an
accident, unless there is a downstairs bathroom.
While being easily accessible for adults, the box
should be out of reach of the children. Another
box should be kept in the car for treating cut
knees on picnics or for anyone hurt in a road
accident.

First aid kits can be purchased but they often
contain more than is needed while leaving out
essential items such as scissors. Assembling your
own kit is cheaper and you can make your own
choice of items. The contents should be kept
simple.

There should be a selection of different sizes of
adhesive plasters with medicated dressing. Sterile
non-adherent dressings which can be bandaged in
position are now also available. Gauze is best
bought in packets so that the dressing is ready for
use instead of having a roll of gauze which requires
cutting. The box should also contain a roll of
adhesive tape for keeping gauze dressings in
place, cotton bandages of varying sizes, cotton
wool, one box of paper tissues, a sling, scotch
tape, scissors, tweezers for extracting splinters
and thorns, and antiseptic lotion such as
cetrimide.

The contents of the box should be checked
from time to time and it must be an absolute rule
that items used up are immediately replaced.

A fresh cut can be protected by an adhesive
plaster dressing. If the edges of the wound are
gaping they can be held together in the correct

position using strips of scotch tape. This method reduces the need for stitching, avoiding both the pain it causes and the mark left by the stitch. Obviously, though, a large cut requires the help of a doctor.

More often, the child arrives home with a grazed knee which occurred some time previously while playing out of doors. There is always the problem of whether to clean the wound. If the blood has already congealed to form the beginning of a scab it is better to leave it alone and only to clean the surrounding skin. This dry scab is the best protection against infection and washing it with antiseptic only softens it, thereby increasing the chance of infection. If practical, leave the graze uncovered by a dressing which tends to make it hot and soggy. Of course the child may demand a dressing as evidence of an honourable wound.

Larger and dirty wounds will need to be cleaned with an antiseptic lotion such as cetrimide before being dressed. The antiseptic can be applied on cotton wool but it is often more practical to use tissues. A roll of cotton wool soon becomes contaminated.

Bleeding can usually be stopped by a dressing applied with pressure. On the rare occasions that an artery is cut, bright blood will come out in spurts. Older first aid manuals used to stress tourniquets and pressure points but tourniquets in unskilled hands are dangerous, and it is impractical to expect most people to know their pressure points. In any case the best pressure point is directly over the damaged artery and the pressure may need to be maintained until the child reaches the nearest hospital.

If the injury occurs in a field where animals have been, there is always the risk of infection with tetanus. This germ can lie dormant for a long time after the last animal left the field. Although the risk of tetanus is slight the only really safe protection is to see that the child's immunisation against tetanus is kept up to date. The initial three shots against tetanus are given in the first year; after this a single shot is needed every five years.

The best first aid treatment for a burnt limb is immediately to put it in cold water for a few seconds. Blisters should not be burst as they protect the burnt area from infection. The burnt area should be covered with a clean sheet and the child taken straight to hospital. Nothing should be put on the burnt area which will stick to it, as this increases the risk of infection – oils, ointments and fluffy dressings must not be used.

A broken arm should be protected by being put in a sling. A broken leg should be bandaged to a splint, which can be a makeshift piece of wood if necessary.

One final but very important point. The child who suffers from repeated accidents is likely to have an underlying emotional problem as the cause. Everyone accepts that the driver who is worried and under stress is more likely to have a road accident. The same situation can arise with children, and the emotional problem is likely to involve the whole family. The statement that a child is 'accident prone' is dangerous since it suggests an explanation for his repeated accidents without looking into the real cause. The situation calls for a professional assessment of the family to see if help is needed.

helping your doctor to help you 13.

Until recently it was the practice for doctors to give orders to parents about the general management of their child, in matters both of health and of illness. The parent would usually accept this 'advice' without question, and the amount of discussion between doctor and parent was minimal. Fortunately, more and more doctors are now coming off their pinnacles, and the medical student of today is being taught to listen to his patients in a way which was unheard of when I qualified thirty years ago.

Helping your child to the full requires a working partnership between parents and doctor, together with the other members of his team, especially the health visitor.

We have already considered the symptoms in your child which should lead you to call your doctor without delay. Now I would like to look at other aspects of the relationship between parents and their family doctor. If it is your first visit to a new general practitioner he will need to ask a number of personal questions which may at first sight seem irrelevant to your child's illness. But the general practitioner of today is a specialist in family medicine, and to do his job properly he must have a clear picture of your whole family and its relationships, together with an idea of your living conditions. He will, for example, need to know a father's occupation, what a mother did before marriage and whether she is still working.

By gathering all this information at the first visit the doctor not only avoids having to find it out on a subsequent occasion but also establishes a more understanding relationship with the new family he is to care for. If on the first visit he fails to learn some of the more intimate family details he may never again be in a position to acquire this information. If the relationship starts off with a brusque, superficial pattern, the doctor will find it much harder to delve deeper on some future occasion when it is needed. It sometimes happens when a child is referred to another doctor that this doctor learns much more about the family than the first one, even though the first one has known the family for years. This happens when the first doctor started off with a superficial professional relationship and has maintained the status quo.

Some doctors are always in a rush – the busy man syndrome. This is seldom the real reason. The good doctor appears to have all the time in the world to listen to his patients, behaving as though you are his only patient that day. The 'busy' doctor may be one who has not been trained to listen to his patients and can only maintain this state by keeping his patients or himself on the move.

Now that, rightly, parents are being taught much more about child health through the mass media, they are able to converse more intelligently with their doctor. They may also use technical words because these now have meaning to them. The use of such terms sometimes causes the doctor to react in a way that suggests he feels the parents are invading his professional territory. It would be unfortunate if this conflict were allowed to continue, because the inevitable reaction of the parents would be either to feign ignorance or to leave the doctor; in either case it is the child who is likely to be the loser.

You should feel free to ask for your doctor's help over the most trivial or the most intimate matters. Your relationship with your doctor cannot be based on fear that he may say you are wasting his time. If you are frightened of cancer or tuberculosis, you should be able to say so without having to have a period of verbal skirmishing with your doctor, when the main point of your visit may be lost.

It sometimes happens that the real basis of your fear is not clear to you. The doctor has been trained to discover what lies behind your anxiety. Sometimes, a doctor is called out at night to see an ill child at home when the parents really want his help over a deep family problem.

You should not be afraid to ask for a second opinion and your doctor should not feel hurt if this happens. Doctors ask for second opinions for their own family more often than anyone else. Not only will the good doctor agree to your request but he is likely to have anticipated that you were losing confidence and therefore made the suggestion in the first place.

With a complete relationship with your family doctor, of the type I have described, it will be obvious that it is always safer to take your ill child to him in the first place rather than to the hospital casualty department. The doctor in the casualty department will not know your child or your family and he will probably be a more junior man than your own doctor. The only exception is the case of an accident or poisoning, when you should go straight to the hospital. But even then it is a good idea, if practical, to telephone your doctor first. He will give you emergency advice and very possibly will telephone the hospital to warn them of your arrival. He will be able to tell the hospital doctor of any important details about your child which will help him in his handling of the situation.

It is interesting to recall that in the old days, when the bulk of the medicines available to the doctor did relatively little good and some did positive harm, the doctor's approach was to prescribe rather than to listen, believing implicitly in the power of his medicine. Today, when doctors have medicines, such as the antibiotics, of a power undreamed-of by their predecessors, the handing over of a prescription is likely to be accompanied by much more conversation between parent and doctor.

14. nursing children at home

The modern approach to the care of sick children, combined with the newer medicines – especially antibiotics – now available means that many more ill children can be nursed at home. Added to this, many operations, for example the repair of a hernia in the groin, which previously meant a stay in hospital of a week to ten days, can be performed on the basis of admission for the day of the operation only.

It used to be feared that children admitted to hospital on the morning of the operation might be given a drink before they arrived, instead of having nothing by mouth for four hours before the anaesthetic. In practice, this risk of a pre-operative drink has been found to be greater in hospital than it is at home. In a busy ward, even when everything possible is done to prevent the child getting a drink, including hanging labels declaring 'nil by mouth' to his bed and to his clothing, a child may get hold of a drink, sometimes from another child. A mother at home can give her undivided attention to the problem.

All this means that mothers will find themselves nursing their sick children at home much more often than in the past. Obviously, this is better both for the child and for his family but mothers need to be taught what is involved. Of course, if any complicated nursing is required the district nurse can come in to explain how to do it but complicated techniques are seldom needed.

The first question is whether he needs to stay in bed. The best answer is to let the child decide. If he wants to be up, it is almost certainly safe for him to get up. There are very few illnesses where bed is essential and your doctor will advise you of them; these apart, recovery is quicker if the child hasn't gone to bed unnecessarily. The idea that a child with a temperature must stay in bed is old-fashioned. A child with a temperature who wants to be up can almost certainly do as he wishes. This means that the child who has been in bed but reached the point of wanting to get up before his temperature has settled is safe to do so.

If your child wants to stay in bed he will probably be happier lying on the sofa in the living room where he can watch you getting on with the housework, rather than being left lonely in his bedroom. This will make it easier for him to watch his brothers and sisters playing even if he doesn't feel well enough to join in. A wise mother will be able to tell when her child has had enough and wants to be put back in his own bed. Being in the living room should also make it easier for him to be occupied by the television.

There are few occasions when it is necessary for a child to be isolated from his brothers and sisters for fear of their catching the same illness. Most infectious fevers, such as measles or scarlet fever, are at their most catching for the day or two before it is realised that the illness is anything more than another ordinary cough or cold. Moreover, the younger children should have been protected against measles by being immunised; this should prevent them getting the illness, or at worst they should only get a mild attack. Scarlet fever is no longer the alarming illness it used to be; it's simply a streptococcal sore throat plus a rash, and it responds very quickly to penicillin.

Talking of measles, there is no need routinely to keep the room dark as used to be done to protect the eyes. The early stages of measles are accompanied by conjunctivitis which may make a child dislike the light. In this case a child may prefer not to be in a bright light. The important point is that if he is happy in ordinary daylight, whether or not he has conjunctivitis, then his eyes will not come to any harm. Measles is a depressing enough illness without making a child feel even more miserable by leaving him in the dark.

Do not make the mistake of overheating a sick child. Doctors today see more sick children suffering through overheating from extra jerseys, extra heaters and closed windows rather than the reverse. Sometimes this causes febrile convulsions. The child should, as always, wear the amount of clothing which makes him comfortably warm and, unless the weather is very cold or foggy, the windows should be open.

The next question is what to give him to eat. A sick child will seldom want any solid food in the early days of his illness, in which case don't try to force him. All he needs is enough to drink and you can choose his favourite one. Adding sugar to the drink is a useful way of giving him some food, and if he will take milk so much the better. The sugar can be ordinary household sugar since this is turned into glucose in the stomach. A lot of unnecessary money is spent on giving glucose.

A child who is not eating will have little solid material for his bowels to open. Don't feel you must make his bowels open for him to get better.

Doctors and nurses should give up the daily ritual of asking patients if they have had their bowels open.

When he wants to eat, choose the foods your child likes best, even if this is fish and chips!

Fortunately, the majority of medicines today can be given by mouth so that painful intra-muscular injections are avoided. These medicines are made to taste nice so that they should not be too much of a problem for the child to take. Tablets can be given with fruit juice or hidden in some jam or marmalade on a spoon. Vomiting is always serious and may make admission to hospital necessary for intravenous feeding of fluids and medicines.

Your doctor will decide when your child is well enough to go outside and when to return to school. These stages can be reached much earlier than was allowed in the past. In general, once a child is running around the house he is well enough to run around in the garden. The timing of his return to school after one of the infectious fevers is laid down by the Department of Health, but quarantine for contacts is now largely a thing of the past.

preparing for a visit to hospital 15.

The chances are high that at some time during childhood your child will have to go to hospital, either for a visit to casualty or to the out-patient department, or for admission to a ward. If you prepare him for what goes on in hospital before he has to go there, his visit will be much less of a surprise or shock.

Obviously, if you are given an appointment to see a doctor in hospital a few days before the event it will be easy for you to explain the reason and what is likely to happen. Even so, speaking as a hospital doctor, I find it surprising how many children I see who have not been sufficiently pre-pared for an out-patient visit. However, it is the emergency admission of children which can be so emotionally upsetting, because the child not only has to contend with the acute illness or accident which has led to his admission but also with the sudden separation from home and being placed in strange surroundings.

There are those who argue that, since an emergency admission is unlikely, there is no reason to explain to children about hospital life. I cannot agree. I believe that the more a child is taught about the ordinary happenings of life the more he understands the world about him, whether or not he actually experiences everything he is told about. Many hospitals now allow children to visit their brothers and sisters, and this provides the perfect opportunity for the healthy children to see what goes on in a ward, and they will probably no longer be frightened of the possibility of having to come in themselves. From talking to children in schools it is clear that it is the sudden accident and subsequent admission to hospital about which they are most frightened.

In the same way, I am always glad to see other children accompanying their brother or sister on an out-patient visit. It takes very little ingenuity on the doctor's part to involve the other children in an enjoyable occasion. They can, for example, not only have the fun of looking into their brother's mouth but can actually help the doctor in getting their brother to open his mouth.

When coming to hospital for an out-patient visit explain to your child that he may have to be undressed and weighed before going into the doctor. There is very likely to be some waiting because the time taken by the previous patient may vary from as little as five minutes to as long as an hour. If the doctor is to see the maximum number of patients in the time available he must allow for some overlap, particularly since patients themselves are often late for their appointments.

If you go to a teaching hospital you and your child are likely to be seen first by a medical student who will then explain his findings to your consultant, his teacher, often with other students present. You should be told of this beforehand but this doesn't always happen, so ask your family doctor if you are not certain whether you are going to a teaching hospital.

A good doctor should sense if it is wiser for you not to talk in the presence of your child, but you are the best judge of this. If you know that you do not want to be overheard by your child, ask if he can wait outside. If you have important questions to ask the doctor which you are frightened of forgetting, write them down beforehand, though doctors sometimes get alarmed by very long lists of written questions.

As much as possible, the doctor in out-patients will arrange for any necessary tests to be done the same day as your visit. This may save both you and him from a second visit. A chest X-ray can often be brought back to the out-patient consulting room for the doctor to see. He will explain to your child that he is going to have a special sort of photograph taken, and he will often show the child the picture when he brings it back with him.

If, following the out-patient visit, it turns out that your child has to be admitted to the hospital ward, the doctor will try not to admit him direct from out-patients, particularly if he is a toddler and, therefore, unable to understand what is going on. Unless the problem is an acute emergency he is subjecting the child to an unnecessary anxiety by immediate admission and is likely to leave him permanently frightened of hospitals. Moreover, since an in-patient admission is likely to be followed by out-patient visits, the child's fear of being kept in is likely to return at each visit. It is much better for you to go home and collect his belongings, returning the next day or later the same day, if necessary. This also gives parents the chance of adjusting to the fact that their child has to stay in.

16. children in hospital

Hospitals are bound to be strange places to a child, but a modern children's ward is far more human than it was even a few years ago. This is unrelated to the premises being modern or not but entirely related to the attitude of the staff. The consultants have the major responsibility for determining this attitude.

Ideally, as I have already stressed, every child should have some idea about hospital before he has to be admitted but this cannot always be the case. It is up to the hospital staff to make life on the children's ward resemble home life as much as possible. This can only be achieved if they look at everything they do through a child's eyes. Admission procedures, for example, can be terrifying if this point is forgotten. In some hospitals, children are still separated from their parents on arrival, so that while the mother talks to the ward sister a strange nurse arrives to take the child off to be bathed. Such thoughtlessness and frightening behaviour should not be allowed. The mother should stay with the child and if a bath is needed it is she who should give it. So much of the ward attitude depends on the training of the nurses. If they have been taught to understand the anxieties of a child and his parents, they will welcome the parents as partners who are helping them to get the child better.

It is seldom necessary for a child to be put to bed on arrival against his will. If he is feeling ill he will want to be in bed but if not it is hardly ever necessary for him to be put straight to bed. When a child is up he should wear his own clothes. It is unnecessarily demoralising for a child to be put into hospital day clothes or to spend his whole day in his pyjamas when he is up and about. Problems involved in wearing their own clothes sometimes arise with toddlers who, because of the frequent changes demanded by soiling, may have their clothes lost in hospital laundry; parents would be wise to take them home to wash.

Visiting for parents should be unrestricted, meaning that they can turn up at any time of day or night. The atmosphere should be such that a mother does not have to report to the ward sister before being allowed to visit her child but just goes naturally to him, greeting the staff as she meets them. On the other hand, when she leaves it is essential she should first tell the senior nurse, as this nurse now assumes responsibility for him in a different way and also has to be ready to comfort him if he is distressed by his mother going.

The mother who wakes in the night at home, wondering how her young child in hospital is, should be free to visit the ward. She should be greeted by an understanding night nurse who does not express surprise at her visiting at such a strange hour.

Unrestricted visiting is a strain on parents and it is up to hospital staff to help individual parents to work out the ideal timing for their particular visit. Parents get very bored by long visits, since just sitting by a child's bed is very different from being active in housework while a child is ill in bed at home. If practical, visits should be short but frequent, a matter of popping in several times during the day if the time spent travelling to hospital is not too great. Where space in hospital allows there should be a parents' rest room, but unfortunately this is often not available.

Whenever possible the mothers of babies and toddlers should be offered a bed in the hospital – whether this is accepted will depend on home commitments. If a mother stays in hospital it is not essential that she should have her child with her in the same room, in fact it may be easier for the mother and for the nursing staff if the mother has a room on her own. When the child is very ill his mother will spend most of the time by his bed, but she can then retreat to her own room for a quick rest knowing that a nurse is continually watching him. There is nothing against a father taking turns at sleeping in the hospital, if he feels like it.

Whenever children are allowed up, they should if possible be allowed outside for walks with their parents. Some hospitals seem to forget to suggest this to parents.

In wards where parents are treated as partners in the care of their children, mothers will be asked whether they would like to say when nursing and medical procedures are being undertaken. Whether a mother stays or not while her child is having an injection or other treatment depends on her, but I am continually being made more and more aware that most mothers can stand anything if it helps their child to get better.

Doctors are divided on the question of visiting a child on the day of his operation. Some refuse a visit until the child is round from the anaesthetic while others involve mothers to the extent of letting them come into the anaesthetic room until his injection makes him go to sleep. It seems reasonable that a compromise should be agreed by all, namely that a mother can remain by the bed while the child goes to the operating theatre and that she is also there when he comes back.

More and more children's wards today employ trained play specialists. Such staff work closely with the doctors and nurses as well as with the parents; they are trained to explain to the staff and parents what the young child is saying in his play. An adult can express his questions and anxieties in words but the toddler may only show it through his play. They are also trained to prepare the children for the different things that will be done to them by using play techniques.

By being more accessible, the staff should be able to answer parents' questions as soon as they arise so that much of the bewilderment and ignorance created by hospital can be dispelled. As a consultant, a useful test is to see whether one can wander through a ward full of parents without being bombarded by questions. The absence of questions is usually an indication that none remain to be answered since staff have already dealt with them.

Parents must be warned that any child, particularly of toddler age, who has returned home from a spell in hospital is liable to feel insecure. This will affect his behaviour so that, for example, he may not dare to let his mother out of his sight, even insisting that he comes into the lavatory with her. A mother who has been warned of this beforehand is better able to tolerate difficult behaviour.

Today's approach to the management of children in hospital should go far to neutralise these bad effects of a stay in hospital. They should in fact go one stage further, and make the experience a gainful one for the whole family.

the value of immunisation 17.

Immunisation is the means by which a child can be protected from catching certain infectious diseases. The child is given an immunising shot so that he reacts by forming antibodies in the same way as he would if he had caught the infection. The number of infections for which such protection is available is growing, though it is still sadly limited, and it behoves every parent to ensure that his children have been given this vital protection. In the United Kingdom routine immunisation is now available against diphtheria, whooping cough, tetanus, poliomyelitis, measles, german measles and tuberculosis. Smallpox vaccination is no longer routine in Britain, but it is required for travel to certain countries.

The immunisation programme varies in different countries according to the needs of the country, being influenced by the incidence of any particular disease. Every programme is a compromise aimed at combining the greatest protection with the least number of shots and the least possible number of reactions.

In the early months of life a baby is protected

by antibodies from his mother which have entered his blood stream while still in the womb. This form of protection is dependent on his mother possessing the necessary antibodies, as a result of having either had the illness herself or being protected against it by immunisation. These maternal antibodies in the baby's circulation not only protect the baby but also reduce the efficiency of the baby's antibody-forming mechanisms, which in any case are not fully efficient in the early months of life. The protection lasts for about six months, so the immunisation programme is usually begun when this period has elapsed. The programme for this country has recently been altered; it starts later than previously and the interval between the shots has been increased. The programme begins with a single shot of 'triple' which combines protection against diphtheria, whooping cough and tetanus. This is given at six months, being repeated at eight months and again at twelve months of age. On each occasion the baby should also receive a dose of polio immunisation given by mouth in a syrup for babies or on a lump of sugar for older children.

This new scheme eliminates the need for a booster dose at eighteen months, this now being given on school entry at the age of five years. This booster shot is against diphtheria and tetanus but not whooping cough, since at this age protection against whooping cough is no longer necessary. At the same time a booster dose of polio is again given by mouth.

Measles immunisation is carried out during the second year of life. A single dose only is required, and it is not given until four weeks after the third shot of 'triple'. Tuberculosis vaccination, using BCG vaccine, is given in this country between the ages of 10 and 13. In countries with a high incidence of TB it should be given to all newborn babies.

German measles vaccination is now available for all girls between the ages of 11 and 13. The reason for this is that if a pregnant woman catches German measles, her unborn baby may be severely damaged by the infection.

It is the doctor's responsibility to check that a child is suitable for each immunisation, and he should always be told of any reactions on previous occasions. In the case of smallpox he will check that the child is free of skin disease, particularly eczema, and that there is no one with eczema in the house to which the child is returning. The reason for this is that the smallpox virus can spread rapidly on skin affected by eczema.

Ideally, booster doses against poliomyelitis should be continued throughout life, at intervals of five to ten years. This is essential for those visiting tropical countries, and in view of the risk of polio in such countries it would be ideal if vaccination against polio were made compulsory for all those who visit them.

Diphtheria immunisation gives complete protection against the disease but it is only by maintaining a high level of immunisation in the community that the epidemics of diphtheria which used to occur in Britain can be prevented from returning. Children immunised against whooping cough may still catch the illness, but much more mildly, and there is therefore far less risk of its serious complications in young children.

Parents should ensure that they have an immunisation record for each of their children. This is particularly essential in the case of tetanus since the treatment of a potentially infected wound differs according to the state of immunisation of the child. If his tetanus immunisation is up to date he is merely given a booster shot, but he may otherwise have to receive a dose of serum (ATS) which can have unpleasant side-effects.

18. the question of X-rays

A mother once wrote to me because her three-year-old son had been taken to hospital with what looked like a badly sprained ankle. The doctor in the casualty department advised against an X-ray because of 'exposure to irradiation' to use his own words. This mother had a daughter of eighteen months who had already frequently been X-rayed for congenital dislocation of the hip, and she was naturally worried about this, particularly as more X-rays would be needed as the girl was still under treatment. The mother was also concerned about the risks to her twin sons, who had been X-rayed a few weeks before their birth, as she had heard of the link between X-rays and later leukaemia.

This mother's concern is very understandable in view of the publicity the subject has received. A doctor has to consider possible risks whenever he orders a test; he must also avoid any unnecessary discomfort to a child and he must avoid needless expense to the National Health Service or to the patient if direct payment is being made.

In the case of a single X-ray of an ankle there is no appreciable risk from irradiation. Clearly, the casualty officer was satisfied from his clinical examination that the foot was not broken. If he had any doubt he would have ordered an X-ray. I imagine that what he meant to convey to the mother was that he was averse to carrying out an unnecessary X-ray, and I would agree with him.

It is clearly essential that the child with congenital dislocation of the hip should have a number of X-rays, but the surgeon in charge would certainly keep these to the minimum. The child would be likely to have a further safeguard: most X-ray departments have a system whereby the dosage of X-rays received by a patient is recorded. If this approaches a dangerous level, because of the number of pictures taken, the doctor in charge is informed. I can remember receiving this information from a radiologist when I ordered a further X-ray on a child who had already had to have several taken.

Needless irradiation of all sorts must be avoided; it is for this reason that the machines in shoe shops, to see the fit of the foot in the shoe, have been removed.

The baby in the womb is at special risk from X-rays, particularly in the early weeks while the organs are still forming. Excessive irradiation of developing organs can cause them to be mal-formed. It is for this reason that the routine chest X-ray of an expectant mother is delayed until after the fourth month of pregnancy, by which time the development of the organs is complete. After this stage of pregnancy the baby's organs grow in size, but development, meaning increase in com-plexity, is complete.

There is evidence of an association between X-rays of babies in the womb and a subsequent increased incidence of leukaemia (and other forms of cancer) among them. This increased risk is relatively small and does not last long, but it is a major reason why X-rays to see the position of the baby in the womb are no longer routine. Because doctors are well aware of this risk, the techniques used and the number of exposures performed are carefully controlled.

It is all a question of calculated risk. The risk to an unborn baby from an abdominal X-ray of his mother exists, even though it is remote. On the other hand, if the information is necessary to determine which way round he is or whether twins are present, the risk to the baby resulting from the doctor remaining in ignorance of these facts is appreciably greater. A baby would be ex-posed to far more danger if his delivery were complicated by unsuspected difficulties which would have been discovered by a controlled X-ray before his birth.

ATTITUDES TO ILLNESS

19. about antibiotics

The discovery of antibiotics has changed the lives of all of us. Are they the panacea for all ills? Why are doctors increasingly reluctant just to hand them out?

When Alexander Fleming discovered penicillin he revolutionised medical thinking. It had previously been thought that any drug strong enough to kill germs inside the body would be bound to harm the body, if not to kill it. The knowledge that a drug could cure an infection soon led to a blind faith in the power of the antibiotics, with consequent tragedies.

It was with chloramphenicol, an antibiotic discovered some time after penicillin, that these dangers were particularly highlighted. Chloramphenicol is a very valuable and powerful antibiotic; it has the disadvantage that in a few patients it acts on the blood-forming apparatus in the bone marrow so as to produce an anaemia which may be fatal. Before this risk was fully appreciated the drug was being handed out for minor infections and in America, in particular, a considerable number of deaths occurred when the drug had only been taken for a cold.

Nowadays, doctors are well aware of the dangers of chloramphenicol so that they take careful precautions when prescribing it, only using it when it has advantages for the patient over other antibiotics.

Of course, antibiotics are only of use against bacteria, whereas the common cold is due to a virus. Viruses are smaller than bacteria, and there is still no drug for routine use against them. But a great deal of research is being undertaken into the discovery of chemicals which are active against viruses, and it seems likely that one of the many promising lines of research will soon produce something effective.

It was in many ways an advantage that pencillin first came into use during wartime, since

54

this meant that its use could be strictly and easily controlled. As a medical officer in the Royal Army Medical Corps, my handling of penicillin was very strictly laid down. All this control meant that the action of this new drug could be rapidly and accurately determined.

Another way in which doctors learnt that antibiotics were not the panacea for all ills was when it was discovered that certain bacteria had the property of being resistant to the action of certain antibiotics. Take penicillin and the staphylococcus, for example. Certain strains of the staphylococcus can produce an enzyme called penicillinase which destroys penicillin. It is as though this particular strain has an extra shield which it can push out to protect itself as soon as it is attacked by penicillin.

These resistant strains of the staphylococcus existed before the arrival of penicillin, but since its arrival they have been encouraged to multiply by a process of self-selection in an environment containing penicillin. In hospital, where penicillin is used a great deal, it is obviously the penicillin-resistant staphylococci which survive, whereas those that are penicillin-sensitive are being killed off every day.

This means that a patient entering hospital for another reason could acquire an infection with a penicillin-resistant staphylococcus which was inhabiting the hospital. This risk would be minimal for a patient being nursed at home and has to be taken into account by the doctor before he recommends the transfer of a patient from home to hospital.

In hospital, the dangerous organisms live mainly on the hands of staff – both nursing and medical – and in equipment containing water. Suction apparatus, infant incubators and baths are all sites where dangerous organisms can collect, to be transferred, therefore, from one patient to another. It is this appreciation of the infectious property of the hands of doctors and nurses which has led to the extreme measures they have to undertake in order not to carry germs from one patient to another. Scrupulous hand-washing between patients becomes a life-saving measure.

At the same time as the greater importance of bacteriologically clean hands has been appreciated, so has the emphasis moved away from the need for masks. Masks prevent droplet infection via the breath but the number of germs transferred in this way in hospital is now realised to be much fewer than was originally thought. A cold or influenza will be passed on by droplet infection, but a doctor or nurse with one of these ought not to allow himself to come into contact with a patient, especially a baby. If he really does have to make contact with a patient then a mask, which was never touched by his hands, would be essential. When the doctor or nurse is well, however, a mask is seldom used except in operating theatres. In most premature baby units, the routine use of masks has now been abandoned. It is possible that in the hot and humid atmosphere of a premature baby unit the wearing of masks actually increases the chance of acquiring a cold.

Fortunately, not all organisms have strains with the ability to resist penicillin. The streptococcus, one of the causes of a sore throat, cannot produce the enzyme penicillinase. This means that it always remains sensitive to the antibiotic. For this reason, a child who has had rheumatic fever is given daily penicillin for the rest of his childhood, in order to prevent any further streptococcal infections which might cause a recurrence of rheumatic fever and consequent rheumatic heart disease. Penicillin is one reason why rheumatic heart disease has become so rare in the United Kingdom, though it is still common in the over-crowded areas of the tropics.

The doctor can discover to which antibiotics the organism causing an infection is sensitive by growing the organism in the laboratory using a special plate containing different antibiotics. Provided the patient is not desperately ill it is wiser to wait to find out which organism is causing the infection and to which antibiotics it is sensitive.

Every family doctor has the services of a bacteriological laboratory to help him. You should feel pleased if, as a parent, he asks you to take your child's throat swab to the laboratory before prescribing any treatment. When you return in two days time to learn the answer you may hear that no harmful bacteria were grown – presumably it was a virus infection. You may be able to tell the doctor that your child is better and both of you will know that the unnecessary use of an antibiotic has been avoided.

the question of handicaps 20.

Any doctor dealing with children, particularly if he looks after newborn babies, is likely to be asked if all the new methods of treating babies, especially those born prematurely, are not increasing the number of children surviving with a handicap. There are no complete statistics to answer this question, but it seems likely that the number of those surviving with a handicap who previously would have died is about equalled by those who previously survived with a handicap but are now normal. The net result is more normal children and an equal number of handicapped children.

The ability to prevent some handicaps and the awareness that babies are being helped to survive, though with a handicap, has focused more attention on the early diagnosis of mental and physical handicap. Medical students today are taught a great deal about developmental paediatrics – an understanding of the normal development of the young child and an ability to recognise, at an early stage, any deviation from the normal.

One problem is that the developmental examination of a baby takes time, and another is that not all doctors have been trained to undertake it.

To ease these two problems an attempt has been made to identify at birth, those babies who have a greater than average risk of developing a handicapping condition. Certain illnesses in the mother render the baby more likely to be damaged in this way and so do problems in the baby at the time of birth, especially lack of oxygen or severe jaundice. The names of those babies who fall into these categories are kept on a special list by the medical officer of health so as to ensure that they are particularly carefully checked for their development. This list is called the 'At risk' register since it is a list of those babies who are at a greater than average risk of a handicapping condition.

It is not usual practice to tell a mother that her baby has been put on this list since this would give her needless anxiety. A mother is told that all babies have checks to see that their development is progressing normally but that babies who have had complications are checked more frequently. It would be natural for the mother to have been told of any complications. When explained in this way no mother will complain that her baby is being checked too often and therefore causing her needless anxiety.

In time, every doctor should have been trained in the developmental assessment of babies. It should then become possible to get rid of the register, since every baby would be receiving the intensive study which today is only possible for those at special risk. Ideally, this routine examination would be carried out by the family doctor rather than by a separate clinic doctor, the family doctor being assisted by a health visitor who is attached to his practice by the medical officer of health.

If a family doctor is not satisfied with progress he will refer the baby to a paediatrician. In all this, the parents will work as partners in the care of their child, being told by the doctors exactly what is going on. In the past, it has been customary not to tell the parents of suspected mental handicap until the diagnosis is certain. I do not believe that parents are best helped by this approach, particularly if their questions about the mental development of their child are fobbed off by answers such as 'It's too early to tell'.

Today's parents want to know the facts, and today's children are best helped by their parents knowing the truth about them. If the doctor's examination of a baby shows him that the baby's development is below average he should tell the parents. This does not involve saying that the child is mentally handicapped, which may well not be the case, but it involves an explanation that a below-average performance may be because it was an off-day for the baby or because the doctor couldn't get the best out of the baby. Obviously, the baby must be examined again after a short interval and most parents will be able to accept and understand this and will only be glad that the doctor is taking so much care.

Early diagnosis of a physical or mental handicap means that the parents can be told the facts about why their child is not doing all he should. This in itself is a form of treatment, since the parents are prevented from the frustration of not knowing the truth and being left in a state in which they are very likely to trail their child from one doctor to another in the hope of getting a favourable report. Early diagnosis also means an early start to treatment which is likely to involve modern play and physiotherapy techniques.

mental handicap 21.

About one child in every hundred born will be mentally handicapped. This major problem and its implications are at last being widely and openly discussed. Unsatisfactory conditions in some long-stay hospitals for such children have highlighted a few of the problems.

In the past, society demanded that many of these children be 'put away' in institutions. This policy of 'social euthanasia' was bad for the children and did not solve the parents' problems. Mentally handicapped children, just like normal children, develop less well when removed from their homes. Early removal from home has an adverse effect on their learning skills and on the development of their personality and behaviour. For the parents, this removal of their child leaves them with guilt feelings that they are not doing all they should for the child. The fact that the child is often not discussed in the family circle only makes matters worse.

The very label 'mental subnormality' only serves to perpetuate the old-world approach to such children. Physically handicapped children are not referred to as physically subnormal and the same should apply to the mentally handicapped. Their needs are the same as those of other children except that they need some things for longer and in greater abundance. Their emotional problems are no different from the emotional problems of normal children except that they are more likely to occur because of the frustrations resulting from being backward and from the way they are handled.

Mongol children are classically described as being friendly, musical and non-aggressive. This is often true, but it is unlikely to be due to an inherent characteristic of the mongol since it by no means holds true for all mongols. It is much more likely that this placid behaviour results from an early acceptance of the child's problems since these are recognised from his physical appearance. The backward child who is not a mongol is likely to have many months or even years when his parents, with ever-increasing anxiety, are trying to make him achieve more than he can. These attempts to make him do better than he is able result in aggressive behaviour in a backward child just as much as they do in children with a normal intellect.

A very small number of disorders causing mental handicap can be prevented by early diagnosis and subsequent special diet. But this does not mean that early diagnosis does not help the large remainder of cases – on the contrary it is essential. First, early diagnosis means that the parents can stop hawking their child round to different doctors, trying to find out what is wrong. Secondly, it means they can begin to be given the long-term guidance which is essential if they are to help their child to the full.

Most parents of mentally handicapped children do not wish to put their child away in an institution and, once they have been told the facts at an early stage and it has been explained that the child's development will be better if he stays at home, very few will demand that he is sent away.

Doctors are unanimous that whenever possible the mentally handicapped child should be cared for at home. But this will only be possible if the family is given maximum support from the community. At the same age that the normal child goes to a nursery school or play group so should the mentally handicapped. More and more play groups for handicapped children of all varieties are being started and there is no harm in mixing normal and handicapped children. The parents of normal children and the children themselves gain by their experience if they mix with those who are handicapped, while the parents of the mentally handicapped are helped to avoid feeling ostracised by society.

For the severely subnormal children there are special schools but many more of these will have to be started to meet the numbers of children involved. These schools are run by the Department of Education and have only recently superseded the Junior Training Centres which were the responsibility of the Department of Health. This is in line with today's realisation that all children, however backward, can learn and therefore should have the opportunity of being taught.

For the less severely subnormal there are special classes, held either in schools for the educationally subnormal or better still in normal schools so that the children can attend the same school as their neighbours.

The potential development of a mentally handicapped child cannot be accurately predicted, but what is certain is that the more he remains in the community instead of being sent to a subnormal community, the better will be his outlook. Mentally handicapped children and their parents need every ounce of support that they can be given by the community to help them with their problems.

22. accidental poisoning

To anyone working in a hospital accident department, one of the alarming changes over the last few years is the increasing number of children who are rushed there after getting hold of someone's tablets in the house or after taking a swig at one of the household cleaning or other fluids left lying around. The greatest danger to the child is that he will die. Fortunately, although the risk is always there, this is not common. But saving the child's life is not the only way of looking at this problem. What are the effects on the child of all that has to happen once he has swallowed a potentially poisonous substance?

Imagine that you have found your toddler with your bottle of aspirins. The bottle is open and he's playing with some of the tablets. You don't know how many tablets were in the bottle and you have no idea how many, if any, of the tablets he has swallowed. Your immediate and very normal reaction is likely to be one of utter terror which, as you rush at your child to remove the bottle, will certainly be transferred to him so that he becomes terrified and bewildered.

What next? Maybe you stick your finger down his throat to try to make him sick and then you rush him to hospital. Possibly you telephone your own doctor who, quite rightly, tells you that the best thing is to go to the hospital accident department as fast as you can. The hospital doctor is faced with the same dilemma as yourself – has your child swallowed a potentially lethal quantity of tablets? He can't afford to take risks so he has to empty the stomach. He does this either by giving a large enough dose of ipecacuanha to induce a violent bout of vomiting or else he gets a nurse to pass a large stomach tube and wash out the stomach. Both of these manoeuvres are unpleasant and frightening.

By now, hopefully, your child is out of danger, but the doctor still can't take any risks. He must keep him in the hospital overnight for observation, in case his condition deteriorates. By the time he comes home to you the next day, even if he has been in the most understanding of hospitals he has been through a very traumatic experience which is bound to leave some sort of mark on his memory. It is this inevitable sequel to that bottle of tablets left lying around which must be used to persuade everybody of the dangers of accidental poisoning if there are children in the house.

What can you do to lessen this risk? Obviously, all poisonous substances must be locked up and the key removed. The medicine cupboard must be high as well as locked since somehow the child may find the key. Ideally, all tablets should be white instead of being attractively multi-coloured like smarties. Some time ago I undertook a research project to determine the favourite colour for sweets, and therefore for tablets, in a child's mind. Red was the most popular but, more important than this, by far the least popular colour was white. I believe this was due to white being associated in a child's mind with a tablet, whereas he associates the other colours with sweets. The difficulty about having all tablets white is the aspect of tablet recognition by colours.

Ideally, as well, each tablet should be individually wrapped in a long cellophane strip which would take a child much longer to undo. Many manufacturers would like to do this but there is the problem of economy and the inevitable increase in cost this would add to the tablets.

Don't leave any tablets loose in your handbag or your drawer and remember, particularly, that the colourful iron tablets which may be so important for a pregnant mother to take are lethal to a young child.

Don't ever take your tablets in front of your child – he may think you are not sharing your sweets with him and hunt them out when you are out of the room. If you have to give your child any pills don't call them sweets in an attempt to get him to take them. His confusion may lead later to accidental poisoning.

Get rid of any tablets left over once a course of treatment has been completed. These should either be returned to the doctor, especially if they are expensive tablets, or thrown down the lavatory.

Household paraffin (kerosene) is one of the most dangerous of the household fluids which your child may find. It can get into the lungs as well as the stomach, causing a fatal pneumonia. It is for this reason that the doctor will not order a stomach washout since doing so would increase the risk of pneumonia. Never put the paraffin into fruit juice bottles – this increases enormously the risk of disaster.

If you have to take your child to hospital be sure to bring the tablets he has swallowed with you so the doctor can identify them and prescribe the appropriate antidote as well as all his other treatment.

Best of all – don't let it happen.

23. physical accidents

I use the term physical accidents to cover all varieties of accident other than poisoning.

Understandably, parents sometimes feel that there is really no way of stopping a determined child from having an accident. Curiosity is evidence of a normal intellect and something to be encouraged; yet this very characteristic is bound to lead him into danger. What can be done to protect him from accidents?

In the first place, the house must be made as far as possible accident proof. Health visitors have been trained in this and are always available to check and advise. Fires must be guarded, electric points must be shuttered and windows protected by bars. Stair rods must not be loose and the head of the stairs should be guarded by a gate while the children are young. It is better to have the dining table covered with an easily washable plastic surface so that tablecloths are never used. It is so easy for a toddler to pull a tablecloth and bring down on to himself a scalding pot of tea. The possibility of pulling a boiling saucepan on to himself should be prevented by having recessed handles. If long-handled saucepans must be used they should be turned so that the handles do not project beyond the edge of the stove.

Oil heaters are far too dangerous to use if there are children in the house. Clothes, particularly nightwear, should be made of non-inflammable material. Pyjamas, for girls as well as boys, should be compulsory since a flowing nightdress can easily get caught in the fire.

The kitchen is the most dangerous room in the house for a young child and yet his mother is bound to spend a great deal of her time there. The safest thing to do is probably to put a play pen in the corner so that a toddler can be safe near his mother, leaving her free to concentrate on her work. I don't like play pens since these are restrictive and not in tune with today's approach to free play for a child, but safety must come first.

Another dangerous room is the bathroom. Cold water should always be run first into the bath so that the bottom of the bath does not become overheated and the risk is eliminated of a child stepping into very hot water. Dangers arise when an older child runs the bath and a younger child gets in first, so the same rules about cold water first must apply to all the children.

Plastic bags will suffocate a child who places one over his head. They should be regarded as deadly poison, being kept out of the house whenever possible and locked up if they really have to be there.

The risk of choking on solid food means that a young child must never be left to feed on his own. Crusts, rusks and large sweets are the greatest danger. If a lump of food gets stuck in his throat, he should immediately be suspended by his feet and thumped on the back to dislodge it.

Children swallow a variety of coins, pins and bits of toys, fortunately without harm on most occasions. It is not my policy to admit such children to hospital for 'observation' until the swallowed object has been passed. I believe that parents can undertake this observation better than strangers and that they are more able to notice any change in their child's appearance or his behaviour indicating the rare complication of intestinal obstruction or perforation. A child who is upset by being in hospital is even more difficult to 'observe'.

Gardens must also be accident-proof and I would plead for no ponds or swimming pools if young children are around. I am appalled by the number of deaths I still hear of caused by a child falling into an ornamental pond.

One of today's problems is high rise flats and their lack of play facilities for the children who live in them. It should be compulsory that all new blocks of flats should contain communal play areas for the children.

Having made the house and garden accident-proof, as far as possible, what next? Children must be trained in safety measures. They must be allowed to explore and must not be so over-protected that they never learn what makes them fall down. Some falls are essential in order to learn how to avoid them.

Although a gate at the top of the stairs is essential for young children, they should be encouraged to learn how to go up and down the stairs with safety. The gate should be left open when a close watch can be kept. Young children should be trained to go downstairs backwards.

For older children, kerb drill is needed to prevent road accidents. The problem here is that the turn left-turn right piece is liable to become a meaningless ritual. A child may unconsciously regard it as an automatic protection, rather like saying his prayers, so that having said his piece he steps off into the road oblivious of the oncoming traffic. The child has to be made to feel responsible for himself and to get away from the idea that adults, being all responsible, are bound to be able to prevent an accident should he forget his safety rules. It helps if the child is sat in the driver's seat so that he can learn the driver's problems about children who dash into the road. Similar lessons are useful when travelling in a bus.

The last major measure to prevent accidents is to ensure normal family stability. As a hospital doctor I am perpetually reminded that children who are admitted with accidents often have an underlying emotional problem. This is one of our commonest ways of learning about a family in a muddle and no child should be discharged from hospital, following an accident, without checking on the family problems and seeing if help is needed.

The adult who is 'in a state' is far more liable to a road accident while driving. The same goes for the child who, if emotionally disturbed, is more liable to every sort of accident. I therefore dislike the term 'accident prone' being applied to the child who has repeated accidents since it suggests the child is at fault, thereby missing the vital point that his accidents are a symptom of a family problem.

After an accident has occurred, emotional problems increase. Parents and child feel guilty and there are liable to be recriminations. The child who suddenly slips from his mother's grasp and dashes into the road to be knocked down and have his leg broken has extra problems. Not only is he admitted to hospital but his leg will need traction involving metal splints, pulleys and weights. I find these among the most disturbed of children but this is understandable. Subconsciously they must feel that not only has their crime put them in hospital but that they are tied down to the bed with weights to ensure they don't escape.

The other group of children with physical accidents who are liable to be very disturbed are those with burns. I think it is even worse for their parents, who so often will be blaming themselves. The child is likely to need nursing in an isolation cubicle to reduce the risk of infection while modern treatment commonly involves exposure instead of dressings. Seeing the burnt area is very traumatic both to the child and to his parents.

24. the recurrent pains of childhood

In all individuals, pain may be due to physical or emotional causes. Physical pain is more easily understood since there is an obvious cause, and because of this it is more acceptable both to the patient and to his relatives. However, even where there is an obvious physical cause, some of the pain felt may be of emotional origin. This is due to 'emotional overlay' and will vary according to the temperament of the individual and his circumstances; it is likely to be greater in the anxious individual than in the person with an even temperament.

Emotional pain may be just as severe as the worst physical pain so that it cannot be excluded by the degree of severity. Diagnosis is made on the basis of associated symptoms and the findings when the patient is examined. In the past there was a tendency for doctors to be trained to diagnose emotional or 'functional' pain, as it is termed, only after exhaustive tests to exclude a physical cause. But the tests and the time taken to carry them out serve only to make the patient more and more convinced of the serious nature of his pain; they may increase the amount of pain felt and, by driving the emotional cause deeper into the patient's mind, make it more difficult to unearth. Today, the early diagnosis of functional pain is stressed in the training of medical students.

Children often develop functional pain and it occurs particularly in one of three sites – the limbs, the abdomen or the head. Very often the mother of such a child will insist that it is a real pain, being concerned lest the doctor thinks the child is making up the fact that he has pain. She is, of course, perfectly correct – emotional pain is just as real as physical pain; it differs in that it arises from the subconscious part of the mind as opposed to the conscious.

'Limb pains' used to be termed 'growing pains' but this is a bad term since the process of growth is not painful. The pain is more often felt in the legs than in the arms, mainly in the thighs and calves. It has nothing to do with rheumatic fever, although this fear is often uppermost in the parents' minds. In rheumatic fever the pain is felt in the joints and these are excruciatingly painful when moved, whereas limb pains are felt in the muscle.

These pains occur more often towards the end of the day and they may wake the child. These facts suggest the possibility of an associated physical cause. Younger children suffer from limb pains more often than older children and it is possible that as they race around all day they put more stresses on their limbs than do older children with their more controlled and better balanced movements. This is not to suggest that any restriction of movement is required for this problem; quite the reverse – no harm will come from exercise. If the child wants to stop for a moment and rub the place where it hurts he can do so but usually when it has been explained to him and his parents that there is no physical disease the pains vanish.

The child with abdominal pains usually points to his navel as the site of his pain. The doctor has to exclude appendicitis and other physical causes but there is usually no difficulty. It is then a matter of explaining to the child that his pains are due to the normal workings of his tummy. With the aid of diagrams it is an easy matter to explain about the intestines and how waves of movement drive the food from the top to the bottom. The child is told that as the food passes along the intestine most of it is absorbed into his body; part of this goes to make him grow and part to act like petrol so that he has the energy to keep on the go. The remainder leaves his body when he goes to the lavatory. In passing along the intestine the food has to go round corners and it is then that the child may feel his tummy working. Anxiety increases the strength of the bowel waves so that the child can be helped to understand the physiological basis to the feelings expressed by adults in phrases such as 'butterflies in the stomach' which they feel at times of anxiety.

The worst thing possible is for these pains to be ascribed to a 'grumbling appendix' since this leaves the parents and the child with the fear that at any moment it will erupt and require an operation. The concept of the grumbling appendix is false; the appendix either roars, producing acute appendicitis, or remains silent because it is healthy.

The child who develops pain in the head as a symptom of emotional stress is usually in an older age group than the child with abdominal pains. Parents often think of eye-strain as the cause of the headaches. Vision must be tested but the cause is much more likely to be due to school problems than to poor eyesight.

With all these children, the doctor excludes a physical cause for the pain at the same time as he is searching out a possible emotional cause. Treatment lies in an explanation to the child and to his parents of the reasons for the pain. In the case of head pains, the emotional cause is likely to lie deeper in the child's mind than it does with either of the other two types of pain.

PART THREE
EARLY COMPLAINTS

25. birth-marks: causes and cures

The good thing about birth-marks is that most of them disappear in time. The odd thing about them is that some are not present at birth!

The most common birth-mark is a flat red mark on the eyelids and sometimes also on the middle of the forehead above the bridge of the nose. There is often a similar mark on the back of the head, in the nape of the neck, near where the hairs stop growing. Since these two pink marks so often occur together they are sometimes called the 'stork's beak' mark since it is there that the stork would have left his mark!

These red stains are made up of capillaries – the smallest of the blood vessels – which are wider than normal. They are sometimes mistaken for bruises and sometimes thought to be pressure-marks made during birth. That could not be true because a pressure-mark or bruise would disappear in a few days whereas these marks do not. However, the good thing about them is that nature has been kind in allowing the mark in front to disappear in almost all the babies, though it may take several months to do so. During the time that it is there a mother will notice that the mark seems more obvious at some times than at others and that crying often makes it stand out. But all the time the front stain is gradually fading away so that it is unusual to see such a mark on the forehead or eyes of an adult.

The stain on the back of the neck is less likely to disappear, but being at the back it does not cause any embarrassment. In fact a lot of people do not even realise they have one. When sitting in a bus or theatre you may sometimes notice the mark on the back of the neck of the person in front of you.

Less common than the stork's beak mark but still very common is the strawberry birth-mark. This is the one that may not be present at birth, especially if the baby is born prematurely. Whether or not it is present on the day of birth, it behaves in the same manner. First of all it gets bigger and then it eventually disappears, so that what may look like a pin-prick at first gradually increases in size and rises above the surface so that it looks very like a strawberry. This process usually takes six to nine months. Then, to everyone's relief, it begins to disappear on its own. The first sign of this is when the colour begins to fade in the centre so that pale islands appear. These pale islands get larger and grow together so that the next stage is a completely pale centre while the rim still remains red. During this time the mark has slowly become flatter and finally the whole thing disappears leaving no sign of where it has been. Occasionally, the skin is left a little whiter than the rest but not enough for anyone to notice.

It was a wise doctor in Plymouth who many years ago first made the important discovery that these strawberry marks disappear. He was looking after both children and adults – before the days of paediatricians – and he said to himself, 'since I don't see these marks in grown-ups surely some of them must disappear on their own rather than all being cut out by the surgeon', as was the vogue at that time. To prove this he had to persuade a number of parents to let him do nothing but watch the mark month by month. This was not an easy task, especially as the marks were getting bigger in the early months. But this doctor was a descendant of the great Lord Lister, the pioneer of antisepsis, and he had the necessary powers of persuasion so that he could eventually watch the marks disappear, much to the delight of the parents who were saved from having an unsightly scar on their children – and not only a scar but one that grew with the child so that sometimes it ended up as an unsightly disfigurement.

A serious type of birth-mark is the so-called port wine stain, often covering half of the face. This may be flat but sometimes its surface is knobbly. The seriousness of this is that it does not disappear on its own and it is often too big for the most skilful plastic surgeon to remove. But all is not lost, thanks to the skills of the modern cosmetic manufacturers. By using a type of pancake base make-up which has been made to match the child's own skin it is possible to camouflage the area. Putting it on may take several minutes every day but it is much better than walking about with a disfiguring stain and being stared at. The use of this make-up need not be confined to girls who have port wine stains, for as it is made to match the child's own skin it can also be used for boys.

Some children are born with moles which may or may not grow hair. Many of these are too small to worry about, especially since they will be hidden away by the clothes. If they are large enough to be disfiguring they are still likely not to be too large for the plastic surgeon who will be able to make a very neat job of their removal.

26. nappy rashes

These are common and distressing both to the parents and to the baby. Much can be done to hasten their cure, and in fact to prevent them, provided their causes are understood.

The common napkin rashes are due to irritation or infection of the skin as the result of its contact, usually prolonged, with urine or stool. Understandably, urine rashes are mainly in the front, being on the insides of the thighs, the genitalia and on the lowest part of the tummy; stool rashes are mainly at the back so that the buttocks and the skin between the legs are most affected.

The most common napkin rash is caused by ammonia and is really an ammonia burn – doctors call it ammonia dermatitis. How is it possible for the baby to be burnt by ammonia when no one has had a bottle of ammonia near him? The answer is that the ammonia has been formed as the result of a reaction between the baby's stools and his urine. Urine contains urea and this substance can be split chemically by the action of certain bacteria which reside in the stools without the baby being ill at all. They are one of the harmless groups of bacteria which live in the intestine.

This reaction is more likely to take place when the stools and urine are left for a long time together in the baby's napkin. The likelihood of this reaction occurring is greater if the baby is being fed on cow's milk instead of breast milk. The stools of a baby fed on breast milk are usually acid which is an advantage since ammonia, being an alkali and therefore neutralised by an acid, is less likely to be formed. On the other hand, the stools of a baby fed on cow's milk are alkaline, and ammonia is thus more likely to be formed.

In the light of all this it becomes easier to work out how to prevent the rash. In the first place, this is another advantage of breast-feeding. Secondly, frequent napkin changes will reduce the opportunity for the chemical action to take place.

What can be done if the rash does occur? The first thing is to recognise ammonia as the cause; this is usually easy because the ammonia may be so strong that a mother's eyes water when she changes the nappies. She will probably say that the baby's urine 'smells strong'. The next thing is to reduce the chance of ammonia being formed by keeping both napkins and skin acid. The napkins should be washed and rinsed in the usual way and then soaked for a few seconds in a weak solution of vinegar, that is, acetic acid. The correct strength is to add one ounce of vinegar to each gallon of water but, to save the bother of accurate measuring, it is usually sufficient merely to add a few drops of vinegar to the water used for the final rinse.

To make the skin acid it is necessary to use an acid ointment. Boric ointment used to be recommended until it was found that it could occasionally cause poisoning if the skin was very raw. Today, a substance called benzalkonium chloride is often used and this is incorporated in some of the napkin ointments on sale.

As far as is practical the child should be left

without napkins. While lying in the cot it may be all right for him simply to lie on a napkin instead of having it pinned round him. Plastic pants increase the liability to napkin rashes by giving the mother an excuse for not changing the napkin as soon as it is wet or soiled. They also make the skin hotter so that it is more liable to become inflamed.

Obviously, the busy and harassed mother wants every possible aid to reduce her work, and plastic pants do reduce the amount of laundry required for bedding and clothes. But she must know their snags. The plastic pants should be loose round the thigh instead of having a tight elastic, and they should be used for as short a period as possible.

The difference in the chemistry of the stool of the breast- and bottle-fed baby accounts for the frequency with which a newborn baby put on the bottle gets a red bottom. It is as though his skin is even more tender at that early age. The chances of this rash developing in a newborn baby who has to be bottle-fed are reduced if his bottom and the whole napkin area are kept well greased. The grease cuts down the amount of contact between skin and urine or stool. The grease used can be something very simple like vaseline or lanoline, or a special 'barrier cream'.

Napkins should be washed only in a pure soap, as a baby's skin is often sensitive to the chemicals used in detergents. Some very nasty rashes have occurred with the new enzyme detergents, and it is best to avoid using these.

27. on allergies

The word allergy is used so often these days that its meaning should be correctly understood. Individuals who are allergic are sensitive to a protein substance which does not affect ordinary people. This protein may be inhaled so that it acts on the lining of the nose to produce hay fever, or on the lining of the lungs to produce asthma.

Alternatively, it may act directly on the skin or be absorbed from the food to act indirectly on the skin, causing conditions such as eczema or nettle-rash.

Allergy can be acquired, and this explains the dermatitis suffered by individuals whose work brings them in contact with substances such as mineral oils, chromium or lime to which they gradually become sensitive. In hospital, nurses can develop skin sensitivity to antibiotics such as penicillin or streptomycin which they are re-peatedly handling in their everyday work.

More often, allergy is inherited from one or both parents. If both parents suffer from an allergic disease the chances of their children being affected are greater than if only one suffers. The common allergic diseases are eczema, asthma, hay fever and nettlerash. The parent does not necessarily pass on the same allergic disease as his own but in passing on the tendency the child suffers from one or more of these diseases. Thus a parent with asthma may give his child eczema; or the opposite may occur. In children, eczema is the earliest allergic disease to appear and since this is most often during infancy it is commonly called infantile eczema. It is much more common in babies who are fed on cow's milk than in those who are breast-fed, so that allergy to cow's milk is probably one factor.

Some children with eczema grow out of the tendency altogether while others, after having it acutely all over as a baby, end up with a chronic form when they are older. This chronic form of eczema appears mainly in the front of the elbows and behind the knees. Some children with eczema develop asthma as they grow up.

Eczema has a fascinating and unexplained re-lationship with asthma in that those children who suffer from both conditions have a see-saw re-lationship between the two disorders. When the asthma is bad the eczema gets better and vice versa. Some children with asthma start each attack with a bout of hay fever, so that sneezing and a runny nose precede the bout of wheezing. It is as though the sensitive substance reaches the nose first and is then breathed down into the lungs where it causes wheezing a few hours later. The runny nose is often mistaken for an ordinary cold so that a mother may describe her child's attack of asthma as being brought on by a cold. But the discharge from the nose in hay fever is clear instead of thick and the 'cold' is not one which passes round the family. Sometimes, an attack of asthma is brought on by an ordinary cold.

In the management of a child with an allergic disorder the doctor has three lines of approach. First, he can try to identify the substance (allergen) to which the child is allergic, so as to remove it from the child's environment. This means taking a very detailed history to discover what brings on an attack. This may be easy, for example when a bout of asthma is brought on by grooming a pony or by stroking a cat. Perhaps the attack of nettlerash has been preceded by eating strawberries or shellfish. Eggs can be a factor in eczema. Unfortunately, it is seldom as obvious as in these examples.

Secondly, the doctor can prescribe what are termed symptomatic drugs, which may prevent the disorder altogether or at any rate reduce the severity of attacks. These drugs include the anti-allergic medicines (anti-histamines) and cortisone. Others, such as ephedrine, dilate the narrowed air tubes in an attack of asthma. The newest drug is disodium cromoglycolate, which is inhaled as a powder and can prevent asthma. More recently it has also been found to prevent hay fever.

The third way the doctor works is to do skin tests to discover to which substance the child is especially sensitive and then to desensitise him to that substance. Skin tests are not much used with very young children but are being increasingly used in children of five years and over. Drops of liquid, each containing one allergen, are placed on the child's forearm and the skin pricked through the drop. A positive reaction is shown by an itching red weal appearing at the site of the prick.

Skin tests are almost always undertaken if the clinical history points to the likelihood of an allergic basis for the disorder – for example, a family history of allergy disease; a seasonal incidence of the disease, particularly with hay fever or asthma; or the onset of asthma in the early morning, suggesting sensitivity to the house mite.

By this means it can be discovered if the child is sensitive to pollens, moulds or other substances inhaled, especially the house mite which is now known to be ubiquitous and an important cause of asthma. Desensitisation involves giving a course of injections, usually eight to ten at weekly intervals, so that the child no longer over-reacts when he next meets the substance.

Desensitisation is most effective if the child is found to be sensitive only to one or two of the test substances. It is not lifelong, so the course may have to be repeated at yearly or longer intervals, depending on symptoms.

Emotion plays a large part in the occurrence of allergic disorders so that even if the allergic cause of asthma is discovered and avoided, an attack can still be brought on by anxiety. The management of allergic illnesses, therefore, requires a balance of treatment between the allergic and the emotional aspects of the child's life and environment.

bronchial asthma 28.

This serious cause of wheezing is on the increase, possibly because of the increased pace of life and its emotional stresses. A typical attack of asthma comes on out of the blue so that the child may rapidly find himself fighting for breath. In older children it may be obvious that the main difficulty is in getting air out of the lungs. This difficulty in expiration is well summed up by the classic remark of an asthmatic patient who said: 'If ever I get rid of this breath I am never going to take another one!' Each long fight to breathe out is immediately followed by sudden inspiration and then another long expiration.

The lung can best be thought of as a series of branching tubes like an inverted tree, each branch ending in hundreds of balloons which are filled with air when we breathe in. The walls of these bronchial tubes contain muscle, contraction of which causes the tube to become smaller. In bronchial asthma there is excessive contraction of the bronchial tubes so that the child has to fight to get air through them.

It seems likely that this tendency to excessive contraction of the bronchial tubes is something with which the child is born, often inherited from one of his parents. Given this tendency, different circumstances trigger off the excessive contraction in individual children. 'Allergy' is one such trigger, indicating that the child is sensitive to a protein substance to which normal individuals are not sensitive. This protein may be inhaled in the pollen from certain grasses or from animal fur or feathers; much less commonly it comes from protein which has been swallowed in the food.

For years it has been known that some asthmatic individuals are sensitive to house dust. Only recently has it been discovered that the major ingredient of house dust to which the individual is sensitive is a minute animal, the house mite, visible only under the microscope. This house mite grows on the scales from human skin and is to be found in bedding, clothes and chair covers. The mite does not have to be alive to cause its effect since protein, to which the individuals are sensitive, is contained in the body of the mite and persists in the dust after its death.

It is possible to test an asthmatic patient to determine those substances to which he is sensitive. The success of desensitisation depends on there being few substances to which the child is sensitive and on a minimal emotional response to frequent injections, since an emotional disturbance is one of the triggers for asthma.

Unfortunately, the effects of desensitisation are short-lived so that the treatment has to be repeated. Greater emphasis must therefore be placed on avoiding those substances to which the child is sensitive. In the case of house dust, much can be done by vacuum cleaning to keep down the amount of dust; this must include cleaning all the crevices in the furniture where dust might accumulate. Damp dusting should be used and only take place when the child is out of the house, as should bed-making.

It is best if hair, feathers and down are removed from the child's bedding in case he is sensitive to any of these. If it is thought possible that the child is sensitive to the fur on one of his pets the animal should be removed for a trial period to see if it makes any difference to the frequency of the asthma attacks.

Fortunately, there is a tendency for asthma to improve as the child gets older. During the period of his life when he is getting attacks it is essential to maintain a good chest shape so that when he stops having attacks the chest is as supple as when he was born. Severe asthmatics are liable to get a serious degree of fixed pigeon-chest. Breathing and postural exercises can be taught by a physiotherapist so that the child learns how to keep his chest in good shape. The child may also find that by doing these exercises and breathing in the way he has been taught as soon as he feels an attack coming on, he can ward it off.

The physiotherapist can also teach parents how to tip and thump the child's chest (postural drainage and percussion) so as to clear from the lungs the phlegm which accumulates during an attack, thus shortening the length of the attack. Children and parents often notice that the initial musical wheeze changes to a rattle as the phlegm accumulates; this change is often described as the onset of 'bronchitis'. This stage can be cut out altogether by using physiotherapy at the right time.

The other value of physiotherapy is that it

gives a mother something positive to do, instead of having to sit back powerless and unable to help her distressed child.

Many new medicines are now available to help treat attacks of asthma and to prevent attacks coming on. Being powerful, their dosage must be carefully adjusted so that the safe limit is not exceeded. If a child has to be brought to hospital in an attack, the name and dose of any drug already given should be known so that the hospital staff can calculate the safe limits for any further doses.

Since emotional factors play such a large part in many children with asthma, any help needed in this direction should be given. No doctor can 'cure' asthma but he can do a great deal to reduce a child's inborn tendency to wheeze, and can perhaps keep it down altogether. Children with asthma should not be regarded as invalids; the attacks should be looked on as a nuisance rather than as a disease and should interfere with everyday life as little as possible.

29. children who wheeze

The word wheeze is used to describe not only the noise made during an attack of bronchial asthma but also any noisy type of breathing of a somewhat musical nature. It tends to be used by parents to cover all sorts of noises which their children make during breathing, so that doctors have to be careful to learn what noise a mother is describing.

One of the most common forms of noisy breathing made by babies is snuffling; this is not a wheeze. Although 'snuffles' are heard during a cold when the baby is unwell, the majority of babies with snuffles are not ill and the noise goes on far longer than would be the case if it were an ordinary cold. In fact, some babies may have snuffles for the greater part of their first year.

The cause of snuffles is to be found in the shape

of the bridge of the nose which in these babies is shallower than usual. For this reason, negro babies often have snuffles. This shallow nasal bridge means that there is less space at the back of the nose for the air passages leading from the nostrils. As the baby grows, the air passages enlarge so that the snuffling noise usually disappears by the first birthday.

Some babies with a shallow nasal bridge have a smaller tear duct for the same reason as they have smaller nasal passages. The tear duct carries the tears from the inner corner of the eye down into the nose. A small tear duct is liable to become blocked so that these babies may get watering from the eyes; the eyes are also more liable to infection, causing a 'sticky eye'. Again, with growth the tear duct increases in size so that the tendency to watering from the eyes and to sticky eyes usually lasts only for the first year of life.

Snoring occurs at any age but in young children is most often the result of enlarged adenoids. Like the tonsils, the adenoids are composed of lymphoid tissue whose function is to protect the body from infection. The adenoids are placed in the midline of the throat at the back of the nose so that they are too high to be seen by looking into the mouth; they are sometimes called the 'pharyngeal tonsil'. When enlarged they may cause sufficient blockage of the nasal passages to produce snoring. The tonsils, if enlarged, are too far forward to obstruct breathing, though occasionally they may obstruct swallowing.

Some of the babies who are described as wheezing are in fact making a gurgling sound in the back of the throat. This may be heard in those bright babies, described as ruminators, who regurgitate their food into their mouths and then chew it over for the fun of it. In the process, some gets spat out, much to the consternation of their parents, whose clothes are stained and smell sour as a result. Similar gurgling may be heard if there is excess salivation, as may happen when a tooth is coming through. It is likely that this noise is a common reason for the oft-repeated statement that a baby cuts his teeth with 'bronchitis'.

Another variety of noisy breathing in young children results from a narrowing of the space between the vocal cords; this is known as congenital laryngeal stridor. This narrowing is due to incomplete growth of the cords before birth. The 'stridor' is heard only during inspiration and it gradually becomes less marked during the first year as the vocal cords grow and the space between them becomes adequate for breathing to be unimpaired. The majority of the babies come to no harm but there is always the risk of laryngitis, usually secondary to a cold, making the space still more narrow. Parents of babies with this type of noisy breathing have to be warned to bring their babies direct to hospital should breathing ever become difficult as well as noisy.

True wheezing is best heard in the child with 'wheezy bronchitis' and in the child with bronchial asthma. Wheezy bronchitis occurs most often in fat, cheerful babies. Although the condition may be distressing, the babies are seldom seriously ill. Antibiotics may be needed but mothers can often best help their baby during the attack by lying them face down on their knees and performing 'postural drainage and percussion'. This technique can be easily taught by a physiotherapist; it involves patting the chest with cupped hands and vibrating the chest so as to loosen the phlegm. The child then coughs it up and swallows it, thereby clearing the bronchial tubes.

Mothers can do much to prevent their young children from getting wheezy bronchitis by not allowing them to get fat. For some unexplained reason, this form of wheezing is almost confined to overweight babies. With the present unfortunate tendency to feed babies with cereals at an early age, the incidence of fat babies and wheezy bronchitis is on the increase.

mouth troubles 30.

Considering the importance of the mouth and how much a child stuffs into it, the amount of trouble it causes is relatively slight. Don't make the mistake of peering into your child's mouth to try to assess the state of his health by the smell of his breath or the colour of his tongue. Bad breath is overrated. It is true that some conditions, such as an acute appendicitis, can be associated with bad breath but the child would be brought to the doctor for vomiting or abdominal pain, not for bad breath. In my experience, it is the anxious mother who complains that her child's breath smells. The child is healthy and my advice is that she should keep her nose far enough away so as not to be able to smell her child. Constipation does not cause bad breath.

The most common infection in a baby's mouth is thrush. This is caused by a fungus called candida; it occurs particularly in bottle-fed babies when the teats and bottles have been inadequately sterilised. White plaques appear on the inside of the cheeks which may look a bit like milk curds. But the difference is obvious – milk curds can be easily wiped away with the handle of a teaspoon whereas you have to rub very hard to shift a plaque of thrush and if you succeed you will make the cheek bleed.

Thrush also coats the tongue white. This is a much thicker fur than the fine white covering produced by milk and there will usually be thrush plaques on the inside of the cheeks as well.

Thrush can be treated with gentian violet, which has the advantage that you can see where the paint has been applied but the disadvantage that it is messy. It causes a sore mouth in a few babies, especially premature ones, so it is seldom used for the very young. Antibiotic drops such as nystatin are an alternative form of treatment.

Throat infection is relatively uncommon in babies. At this age the tonsils are very small so the whole of the throat becomes inflamed if it does occur.

In young children of the pre-school age an acute attack of mouth ulcers is common. This is usually due to a virus called herpes simplex which has reached the child from someone, usually a close relative, who gets cold sores round the edge of the mouth. The sores are due to the same virus and the individual who gets them has usually had one attack of mouth ulcers in childhood. This produces enough immunity to prevent another similar attack but it is not strong enough to rid the body of the virus altogether. The virus continues to reside in the mouth, producing cold sores when the body's resistance is lowered, for example by a cold. The sores are the result of the cold, not the cause of it. The parent who gets cold sores is likely, therefore, to pass the infection on to his child, giving him one attack of mouth ulcers and a subsequent liability to the same sores.

The virus is not destroyed by antibiotics but mouth ulcers always clear up on their own in about ten days. They are very painful and this is made worse by applying paints to try to make them heal quickly. For this reason, I do not give any special treatment; I merely encourage the child to drink, partly because his body needs fluids and partly to keep the mouth moist. He will not be able to eat solids in the early days and this does not matter.

A different condition is the single mouth ulcer which, unlike the herpes virus ulcers, tends to recur. It may be on the inside of the cheek or on the gum. Its cause is unknown but since it can be due to dental trouble it is wise to visit the dentist. Cortisone ointment is often prescribed but if this is not available any greasy ointment such as vaseline will relieve the pain. By coating the ulcer the grease protects it from being rubbed.

'Tongue tie' is a non-starter as a mouth trouble. The fraenum, which attaches the tip of the tongue to the floor of the mouth, may be short or long but it does not matter which. In either case the child will be able to stick out his tongue like everyone else when he gets older because it is the front part of the tongue which grows most in children. 'Tongue tie' does not cause speech or feeding problems; there are very few doctors today who would recommend cutting it.

I have not included 'teething' here. It is a very exaggerated cause of trouble; for a general discussion of teething see page 103.

eye troubles 31.

In the very young baby the most common trouble is a 'sticky' eye: a yellowish-white discharge from one or both eyes makes the eyelids tend to stick together. In general, the earlier it occurs the less serious is the problem. A sticky eye on the first or second day of life is usually due to irritation from blood and amniotic fluid getting into the baby's eyes during birth. This is a chemical form of irritation rather than an infective one. To prove this requires the examination of a bacteriological swab which the doctor always needs to take. The fact that this test nearly always shows no evidence of germs is my reason for believing the problem to be due to a chemical irritation.

There is no need to wait for the result of the test before starting treatment. The eyes require bathing at frequent intervals in order to wash away irritating matter. This can be done with cotton wool soaked in a salt solution. However, although it is traditional to use a salt solution (one teaspoon of salt to one pint of water), it is perfectly all right to use tap water. Each eye is bathed from the inside corner outwards; this direction is used to reduce the chance of carrying debris from one eye across to the other. For the same reason, a baby with one sticky eye is nursed on his side with the affected eye next to the mattress. If the bad eye were on top, debris could flow over the bridge of the nose and enter the good eye. In hospital, a more efficient method of bathing may be used. By attaching blood transfusion tubing to a bottle of sterile salt solution a jet of the fluid can be directed on to each eye in turn so as to wash it clean.

After the first two days of life the occurrence of a sticky eye is likely to be due to an infection which the baby has caught after birth. This is usually caused by a staphylococcus germ which may also be responsible for causing infectious spots on the skin and infection of the navel, giving it, too, a sticky discharge.

In previous days, gonorrhoea was a common cause of infection of the eyes of newborn babies, with grave risk of subsequent blindness. Fortunately, penicillin treatment of pregnant mothers with gonorrhoea has reduced this risk but the rising incidence of gonorrhoea has made doctors very aware of the renewed possible risks to the eyes and sight of newborn babies. Scrupulous antenatal care is vital.

Some babies get repeated bouts of sticky eye, often in association with persistent watering from the eye between bouts. This is usually due to complete or partial blockage of the lacrimal duct which carries the fluid in tears from the eye into the nose. This channel is the reason for sniffing by someone who is crying; the extra tears would fill the nose and come out in front, if it were not for this.

Fortunately, blockage of the lacrimal duct usually clears itself in the first few months of life. It is, therefore, the usual practice to do nothing but bathe the eye until about six months of age in order to give the channel time to clear itself. If the blockage still persists, an eye specialist can easily clear it by passing a very thin probe down the channel while the baby is anaesthetised.

A potentially serious problem in babies is a squint – sometimes called a lazy eye. This does not matter for the first two to three months of life, before the baby has learnt to use both eyes together. At rest, the eyes diverge, and before normal synchronous vision has been achieved with both eyes, a baby may look cross-eyed at times as a result.

After the age of three months a squint must always be taken seriously. It is usually due to imbalance of the muscles which move the eye and it causes the baby's brain to see two images. The brain then subconsciously suppresses one of these images; suppression of the image from one eye leads to blindness in that eye from disuse in a relatively short time. An eye specialist should see every baby who is still squinting at the age of three months, but they should be seen earlier than this if the squint is obvious and persists throughout the day. Proper treatment will prevent future blindness.

A squint which does not develop until a child is about three years old is usually due to an error of refraction. The child is either long- or short-sighted and he has to squint in order to see properly. The provision of glasses of the correct strength to restore normal vision removes the need to squint.

tonsils and adenoids 32.

Why do we have tonsils and adenoids? They are composed of lymphoid tissue and their job is to guard us from infection. Being sited in the throat and at the back of the nose, they form one of our first lines of defence against germs entering the body by this route.

During the first year of life the tonsils and adenoids are always small – acute tonsillitis is rare in young babies. During childhood the tonsils and adenoids increase in size in common with the rest of the lymphoid tissue throughout the body. This increase in size also affects the lymphatic glands which are part of the same system, and these can often be felt in the neck of a young child. Mothers often worry unnecessarily about 'glands', being unaware that their increase in size is normal.

By the end of childhood the tonsils, adenoids and lymphatic glands become much smaller. It is believed that this natural increase in size during childhood is related to the fact that acute infections are most common during this period, thus requiring the strongest defences.

During an attack of acute tonsillitis the tonsils become acutely inflamed and therefore swollen. This is not an indication for their removal. A boil on the back of a child's hand causes swelling but no mother would dream of asking for the hand to be removed because of this; however, she will often make this remarkable request in relation to large inflamed tonsils.

The large size of the tonsils is seldom, if ever, an indication for their removal. Large tonsils are actively carrying out their job, whereas those that have become small from scarring due to repeated infections may need to be removed. Large tonsils do not obstruct breathing but occasionally obstruct swallowing; however, one is much more often surprised by those large tonsils which have no effect on swallowing.

Large adenoids are liable to obstruct breathing so the child has to breathe through his mouth. But the mistake should not be made of regarding the child who has the habit of keeping his mouth open as being a 'mouth-breather'. The majority of such children will be found, on testing with cotton wool held in front of the face, to be breathing through the nose.

The most serious effect of large adenoids is to increase the liability to inflammation of the middle ear, since when enlarged they block the opening of the Eustachian tubes which leads to the middle ear. Inflammation of the middle ear must always be treated seriously as it can lead to deafness. Consequently, a doctor may recommend removal of adenoids in a young child who has had one or two attacks of middle ear inflammation.

Removal of tonsils may be recommended in a child who has repeated attacks of tonsillitis. It is seldom necessary before the age of four years, and in coming to a conclusion the doctor and surgeon will want to study the child between attacks to assess his general state of health. They will be more influenced by the child as a whole than by the appearance of his tonsils. Mothers would therefore be well advised not to try to assess the health of their children by peering down their throats.

wind and colic 33.

It would be interesting to discover when the present emphasis on bringing up the baby's wind first began. The importance of 'winding' the baby has certainly been strongly emphasised in this country since Victorian times, and in America the need to 'burp' or 'bubble' the baby is similarly advocated. But this attitude to wind is by no means universal. It is not a feature of native mothercraft in developing countries, though it is now practised by the educated classes in such countries. Even in developed countries it is not a universal practice: a Czechoslovakian lady married to an Englishman had her first baby in England and was duly taught the ritual of winding the baby. She had her second child in Czechoslovakia, where they don't have 'the wind', so that when, in the hospital, she began to rub and pat the new baby's back to get up the wind the doctors, nurses and mothers all asked her what on earth she was doing to her baby.

In the early months of life, when it is so difficult to understand a baby's behaviour and his feelings, crying is commonly ascribed to hunger or to wind, depending on whether or not he has recently had a feed. The fact that he draws his legs up while crying is used as evidence that the cause of the crying is 'the colic' although this movement naturally occurs whenever a baby cries. While crying, the contraction of the abdominal muscles may force the baby to pass wind from the back passage; however, instead of accepting this simple mechanical reason for the passage of wind, mothers are liable to turn it the other way round and say he was crying because he wanted to pass wind. When the baby is soothed by his mother the valve at the upper end of the stomach relaxes so that he is likely to bring up wind. Again, this is used as evidence that the crying was due to wind.

We have no difficulty in recognising fetishes in other cultures, for instance the provision of charms to be worn by some children in developing countries in order to ward off the evil spirits; we must also recognise our own fetishes, being aware that the present-day obsession with bringing up the wind has become comparable to a need to get the evil spirit out of the baby.

Of course babies, like adults, swallow air during feeds, so that an X-ray picture of the abdomen which shows up the air results in an exactly similar picture in both age groups. But no one feels the adult must be made to bring up his wind.

What then should the mother do? At the end of the feed she should cuddle and play with her baby in her arms; if during this time he brings up wind then she can tell herself that there was some wind ready to come up. If, on the other hand, no wind is brought up she need not feel that she cannot lie him down until it arrives. She should lie him down when, following his feed and his cuddle, he has become dozy and obviously ready for sleep.

If only wind made no noise when it was brought up perhaps mothers would feel differently. Mothers have been attuned by grandmothers and books to derive enormous pleasure from the noise, so that eventually their whole regime with the baby may become centred on waiting for the burp.

It should now be obvious that gripe water is a waste of money. Some families should be able to save a tidy sum for useful expenditure on something more useful.

Where does 'three-month colic' fit into this concept? The term is used for babies who, during the first three months, draw up their legs and scream, most often in the early evening between 5 and 7 p.m. In working out the causes of this common problem it is essential to consider why the very young should be particularly involved and why in the early evening. The young baby is much affected by his surroundings and the atmosphere around him. At the same time, he has not yet reached an age when he can take evasive action either by walking away or by behaving in the negative way so often adopted by toddlers. The other point to consider is why this problem so often occurs in the early evening. Is anything special happening to the baby at that time? Clearly, the answer is yes – this is the busiest time for his mother, when she can give the least time to her baby and when she is likely to be at her lowest ebb. She is rushing through her baby's routine which may include a 6 p.m. feed and putting the other children to bed in order to get the house straight and the meal ready for her husband's return from work.

If three-month colic is understood in these human terms rather than being explained on the usual mechanistic lines, its solution becomes simpler and more effective. The baby needs unhurried attention, not anti-colic medicines. Father's help must be enlisted so that he tries to get back earlier from the office, the 6 p.m. feed perhaps becoming the one meal in the day which he is lucky enough to be able to give to his baby.

the baby who vomits 34.

Vomiting is such a common problem with babies that mothers need guidelines to know how to deal with it, and particularly whether to regard it seriously.

The best way to decide how seriously to regard the vomiting is whether the baby seems ill. Large numbers of babies, aged 6 to 12 months particularly, vomit for the fun of it. They do it as a habit which they clearly enjoy. Such babies are not ill – in fact they are unusually happy and cheerful. But every time they are picked up they are found to be lying in vomit so that their clothes smell. More than that, they vomit over their parents' clothes so that fathers will not pick them up or they hold them at arms length in order to avoid damage to their suits. Little pools of vomit are left on the carpet where they cause permanent stains. However, despite the smell and the apparent large quantity of vomiting the baby is happy, thriving and gaining weight.

All babies enjoy their mouths once they have been discovered, usually around the age of 2 to 3 months. It is then that they start to cram their fingers into their mouths; this is for exploration and nothing to do with teething. These vomiting babies derive a greater than average pleasure from their mouths so that they may be seen to regurgitate their food back into the mouth from the stomach and then to chew it over, like chewing the cud. This is called rumination. In the process of chewing, some of the regurgitated milk and food is spilt out of the mouth causing smells and stains.

Mothers of such babies put all their efforts into trying to stop the vomiting, believing it to be harmful to the baby. But since the baby is thriving and happy he is not coming to any harm and therefore there is no reason to stop the habit. In fact it would be very difficult to do so because it is such a strong habit.

All that needs to be done is to explain that the baby is well, leaving it to his mother to take what steps she can to reduce the damage to clothes and carpets. The mother of such a baby will often arrive to see her doctor armed with a cloth or tissue with which she keeps dabbing the baby's mouth. This tends to encourage the habit since it merely adds to the pleasure he derives from his mouth.

One compensation is that these babies are usually bright. They are extroverts who often cry less than the average. I have sometimes wondered if their extrovert nature and the pleasure they derive from their mouths will lead them to a career involving public speaking. Perhaps some become politicians!

Quite different from these thriving babies is the baby who suddenly vomits for the first time, particularly if he looks ill. The serious causes of vomiting are obstruction in the bowel and infection anywhere in the body. Both produce additional symptoms to the vomiting so that there is little difficulty in separating them from the cheerful thriving vomiters already described. The babies look ill, and in the case of bowel obstruction the abdomen may become swollen. In the case of infection the baby goes off his feeds – always a serious matter. A change may occur in the baby's cry: obstruction causes the baby to have bouts of screaming and, instead of going red in the face as is usual when crying, the baby goes pale during the bout; the baby with infection is often miserable with a continuous whimpering cry quite different from his usual noise.

Obviously, whenever a mother is in doubt about the seriousness of vomiting in her baby she must call her doctor, but these guidelines should help in her decision whether or not to do so.

threadworms 35.

In temperate climates, such as Britain, the threadworm is the most likely variety of worm to be present in a child – and not only in children but in their parents as well. How much trouble do they cause and is it necessary to try to get rid of them at all? These are the questions asked by parents.

The threadworm is well named, being whitish, about an inch long and looking like a thread of cotton. For a short time after being passed with with the motion it can be seen to wriggle about. Parents, understandably, feel disgusted by the idea of their children passing a living worm and it is this disgust and distress which causes many of the symptoms.

To know more about these common worms and how to deal with them it is necessary to know something of their life-cycle. The worms live in the large intestine, this being the lower part of the bowel. The fertilised female worm emerges through the back passage to lay her eggs on the surrounding skin and does this mainly at night. This causes irritation so that the child scratches his bottom and contaminates his hands with eggs. These eggs, visible only under the microscope and not to the naked eye, are then likely to be transferred to the child's mouth when he sucks his hands or bites his nails. They may also be passed to other children from hand to hand.

Although abdominal pain is often thought to be a symptom of threadworms, this is rarely the case, since the worms live peacefully in the intestine. Sometimes an appendix removed for acute appendicitis is found to be full of threadworms but this does not necessarily mean that the worms caused the appendicitis since the appendix is their favourite home. The association of abdominal pain and threadworms is more often due to emotional causes, being a reflection of the parents' and often the child's own feelings of disgust at seeing the worms.

The direct symptoms caused by the worm result from irritation around the back passage. This may cause sleeplessness and, sometimes, bed-wetting. Occasionally, in a girl, the worms enter the vagina, setting up inflammation and causing a discharge.

To help the doctor make his diagnosis it is best to bring the worms in a pot when visiting him. If this is impossible the doctor will probably be able to make the diagnosis from the description given. He may, however, choose to do a simple test: a piece of Scotch tape is placed across the back passage first thing in the morning before washing and before the bowels have been opened; any eggs lying on the skin become stuck to the tape which is immediately removed and examined under the microscope for the presence of eggs.

In the past it was sometimes suggested that the worms were so common and the trouble they caused so slight that treatment was unnecessary. This suggestion was influenced by the messy nature of the treatment, which in those days consisted of gentian violet capsules taken by mouth. If the capsules were bitten the violet dye mixed with saliva was to be found everywhere. In any case the stools became violet and any incontinence led to permanent staining of clothes and sheets.

Today, treatment is simple. New drugs, particularly piperazine, are easy to take and with some preparations a single dose only is required. This medicine should be taken by all members of the household, adults as well as children, since symptomless infestation is common; if one member of the family is left untreated he could re-infest the rest. As well as giving this medicine, steps should be taken to prevent the child from transferring eggs from his bottom to his mouth. The life-cycle of an individual worm is only six weeks, so if re-infestation of an individual is prevented for that time all the worms will have died out.

To prevent this transfer, the child's nails should be cut short to reduce the chance of eggs being trapped under the end of the nails after scratching. Tight pants should be worn at night to prevent contact between finger and bottom. An additional precaution is to smear a mercury ointment around the back passage; this deters the female worm from emerging to lay her eggs and she is therefore passed with the next motion.

Threadworms, therefore, are common but they seldom cause serious symptoms. They do not cause loss of weight. However, since treatment is simple it should always be given to all members of the household.

36. hernia in babies

A hernia is the technical name for a rupture. These are common in babies, particularly at the navel but also in the groin. The result is a lump, containing intestine, which has been pushed through a weak place in the muscular wall of the abdomen.

The umbilical hernia which occurs at the navel is extremely common. It becomes more obvious when the baby cries, so that mothers, understandably, think it is the lump which is making the baby cry. In fact it is the other way round: crying causes the abdominal muscles to contract, thus forcing the intestine through the rupture, if there is one. When crying stops the intestine slides back into place again.

Although the umbilical hernia looks alarming when it is stretched in this way, there is no cause for alarm; it almost always disappears on its own without any treatment. Sometimes it takes as long as four or five years to disappear but, provided they are left alone for long enough, very few need to be treated by a surgical operation.

It used to be common practice for such navels to be strapped in order to hold them back, but most doctors stopped doing this when a study of a large number of such babies showed that natural healing could be delayed by strapping. Free movement of the abdominal muscles is needed for natural healing of the umbilicus.

The rupture in the groin is called an inguinal hernia. It occurs much more often in boys than in girls. During intra-uterine life the testicle first develops inside the abdomen; it then passes down a canal in the groin to reach the scrotum. This canal should close once the testicle has passed through, but occasionally it fails to do so. Should it remain open a small loop of intestine can pass through into the groin and sometimes go on into the scrotum. The intestine can be pushed back and often goes back on its own when the child lies down. Coughing makes it more obvious.

The inguinal hernia differs from the umbilical hernia in that it can be dangerous for the baby because of strangulation. If this occurs the lump becomes hard and painful, and can no longer be pushed back into the abdomen. Lack of blood to the piece of intestine caught in this way can cause serious damage.

Because of this risk of stragulation, which is greatest during the baby's first year of life, it is now usual for the surgeon to operate within a few days of the hernia's first appearance in order to repair it. A strangulated hernia, of course, requires an immediate emergency operation.

In view of the complicated descent undergone by the testicle during development, it is not surprising that this descent is sometimes incomplete. Fortunately, the vast majority of boys with one or both testicles undescended have what is termed a retractile testicle. The organ has been drawn back into a pouch immediately above the scrotum and can be milked down into the scrotum by a doctor. This requires a warm room, warm hands and sometimes quite a bit of patience. However, provided this can be achieved, the testicle is sure to come down on its own by the time of puberty and no operation is necessary.

It is part of the routine examination of the newborn baby boy to check that the testicles have descended properly. If they were not felt at birth the doctor would normally arrange to check again in a few days because with some babies, especially those born prematurely, the testicles may descend shortly after birth. If one or both was still absent the doctor would usually arrange to check again when the boy was two or three years old.

The operation to bring down an undescended testicle is now usually carried out between the ages of four and five. By this age the testicle will rarely come down on its own and it has to be correctly situated in the scrotum for full function when the boy grows up. It is a relatively simple operation but, like every other procedure, must be explained to the child before he goes down to the operating theatre to be anaesthetised. Even very young children can be helped to understand the need for such operations provided the adult is not embarrassed and can see the problem through a child's eyes so that his explanation is simple.

An inguinal hernia and an undescended testicle sometimes occur together. Immediate operation is required for the hernia, and at the operation the surgeon will place the testicle in the correct place. If he left it until later the scar from his first operation might make it impossible.

PART FOUR
FORMING HABITS

37. why do babies cry?

A certain amount of crying is normal for all babies in the early weeks of life. The duration of this normal crying varies with each baby but averages about two hours within the twenty-four. The baby's first cry, as soon as he is born, is essential for his survival, ensuring adequate expansion of the lungs so that the brain immediately receives oxygen from outside now that the supply from inside, through the afterbirth, is cut off.

For the first few weeks of life a baby's cry is his only positive reaction to his environment, so we would be wrong to try to explain it in the same terms as are appropriate for the older child. In the past, doctors and nurses as well as parents have tried to find an explanation in mechanical terms, such as 'the wind' and 'colic', but this is unhelpful as well as probably being inaccurate. Mothers will find looking after their babies much more interesting if they look further in trying to understand their behaviour.

The newborn baby has strongly developed 'righting reflexes' so that when placed on his back on a flat surface his arms and legs fly out in a standard pattern. This always makes him cry but the crying can usually be stopped by placing your hands on his trunk and limbs so as to stop him rolling about. It is for this reason that babies in cots are quieter when tucked up tight, and it is probably because of this effect that swaddling clothes evolved. In countries where the baby is carried on his mother's back a similar cloth for wrapping round is used.

Hunger is a strong stimulus for crying, thus ensuring that the baby is not left to starve. However, because this is such a real and well-known cause for crying the mistake is often made of ascribing all crying to hunger. This may lead not only to over-feeding but also to a failure to understand the young baby's developing needs. A baby will cry from boredom when he needs stimulation and play. Even a very young baby will cry more if his mother is upset, since he is able to sense his mother's feelings and tensions.

Crying does not result from something wrong in the mother's milk, yet thousands of babies have been weaned for this belief. Possibly there may not be enough breast milk but this is quite a different matter. Strangely enough cow's milk seldom gets blamed in this way.

A wet or dirty napkin is frequently described as the cause of crying but probably this is seldom the cause. It is true that a baby may cry because he is cold but the soiled napkin is likely to be warm rather than cold. This is an example of the adult projecting the feelings she would expect from herself when trying to understand a baby's behaviour.

Pain such as that a baby feels when he has an injection or vaccination will evoke a short sharp cry which in young babies is immediately forgotten. It is not until over the age of six months that such incidents are remembered, causing the baby to cry when the needle is produced again.

Many mothers returning from hospital are disturbed to find how much their babies cry, particularly if they have been told that their baby is quiet at night. Such mothers are liable to feel guilty that they are bad mothers, whereas the truth is that busy nurses hardly notice a baby crying.

Teething is not a cause of crying; if it were, we should expect individuals to be crying from six months until about twenty years of age! However there is always a reason for a baby crying and the more a mother learns to understand her baby the more quickly will she be able to determine the cause of his crying.

the truth about teething 38.

Why has teething been regarded as the cause of so many of the things that seem to be wrong with the baby in the second half of his first year of life? The first tooth, a central incisor, usually appears at about the age of six months. Up to that age there has been nothing concrete to blame for unexplained symptoms. 'Wind' and 'colic' are the popular explanations but even to those who believe in them (and I certainly don't) they are difficult to see. How do you measure the amount of wind a baby brings up? Should you be recording the loudness of the burp? It is even more difficult to measure the amount of wind he has left in him, particularly when you remember we are all full of wind.

Into this ethereal atmosphere arrives the first tooth. No wonder all those unexplained symptoms, particularly his crying, have at last something obvious as a peg on which mothers can hang their worries and beliefs.

Of course, to ascribe many aspects of a baby's behaviour to 'teething' does no harm, but there is a very real danger in this which worries doctors. If a baby goes off his feeds at the same time as a tooth is coming through, and after the age of six months the chances are high that this will be the case, his mother is very likely to decide that the tooth is the cause of the loss of appetite. This overlooks the early stages of an illness, particularly an infection, which is the most likely cause of his loss of appetite.

Babies do not localise symptoms to the same extent as adults, so that a sore throat or an infection in the urine fails to produce the local symptoms found in older children and adults; babies merely go off their foods. It is the doctor's job to locate the infection, but the mother must first take the child to the doctor instead of diagnosing teething and possibly giving treatment herself. Every year I see several babies with serious infections brought up late because their mothers thought the symptoms were due to teething. Another dangerous belief is that teething causes convulsions; this is never true.

After all this, what can we put down to teething? The eruption of teeth in most children is not accompanied by any symptoms. Most of the village mothers in developing countries have not even heard of our sort of 'teething'. Certainly it doesn't make a baby burst out crying, although some babies may be a bit miserable and moan a little. The cheek on the same side as the erupting tooth may become pink and the gums red and swollen.

Many mothers say their children cut their teeth with 'bronchitis'. Mostly they are describing the coughing and gurgling which results from the extra saliva produced in response to the eruption of a tooth.

If symptoms really are due to the discomfort caused by an erupting tooth what can a mother do? In the old days she would give a teething powder and since these usually contained mercury the child sometimes got 'pink disease' from mercury poisoning. Today, it is illegal to put mercury into teething powders so that the substances they contain are innocuous even if they are unlikely to be of any benefit. Doctors will sometimes prescribe a junior aspirin or safer still paracetamol if a soothing medicine is really required.

Teething, therefore, is something which happens in most babies without causing any trouble. There is a great deal of truth in the saying that teething only produces teeth. The danger lies in ascribing symptoms to teething and over-looking more serious causes such as infection. The only safe approach is like the old Shell advertisement in which, as a car hurtled past, the comment was made: 'That was Shell, that was'. In the same way, teething should only be diagnosed when the symptoms have disappeared and a tooth has come through. It is then safe to say; 'That was teething, that was'.

thumb-sucking 39.

Why do babies suck their thumbs? Is this some-thing harmful and should mothers try to stop it? How often one is asked this question.

FORMING HABITS

Thumb-sucking is a natural phase of development through which most children pass, although a few miss it out all together. There is evidence that babies occasionally suck their thumbs while still in the womb, but more often it starts during the first few weeks of life; a baby who has not started to suck his thumb by his first birthday is unlikely ever to do so. Babies vary enormously in the amount they suck their thumbs or fingers and this variation is related to individual sucking needs and the amount they are satisfied. It is believed that suckling at the breast satisfies this need more than sucking on a bottle. Suckling involves a pumping action of the tongue which draws the nipple far into the mouth, the tongue and lower lip always being in contact. At the same time, the lower jaw moves backwards and forwards. Sucking from the teat of a bottle is different since suction, as opposed to suckling, uses the cheek pads. It would be interesting to discover the total length of time babies spend thumb-sucking if brought up in a developing country with easy access to the breast, and to compare this with babies from the same country brought up on the bottle. If these theories are correct the bottle-fed baby would thumb-suck for longer.

A different aspect of thumb-sucking is that it allows the child to explore his mouth and learn more about his own body. Modern physiotherapists, when treating spastic children who cannot put their thumb in their mouth, will teach them to do so in order that this experience is not missed. To my mind the strongest argument against a dummy is not its dirtiness but that it prevents the child from exploring his mouth with his fingers.

Seen in this light, there is no reason for mothers to pull the thumb out of the mouth, a manoeuvre which only frustrates the child, particularly if he is physically restrained from getting his thumb into his mouth.

At the start I explained that thumb-sucking was a phase of development through which most children passed. The usual period for this phase is approximately the first year of life. The child who continues the habit after this is using his thumb as a comforter, particularly when he is frightened or going to sleep. Some children who have lost the habit regress to this infantile behaviour when admitted to hospital. Boredom can also cause perpetuation of the habit so that the child who is left for long periods in the pram is more likely to continue his thumb-sucking than the child who is stimulated to play and will probably forget about it. Obviously, the right way to deal with the child who continues to thumb-suck beyond the usual age is to deal with his insecurity or boredom rather than directly attacking the thumb.

Fortunately, damage to teeth will not be lasting if the habit is lost before the permanent teeth start to come through at the age of six years.

dribble . . . dribble . . . dribble 40.

A mother once wrote to me saying that her three-year-old son dribbled copiously and had done so since he cut his first tooth. She had been told by her dentist that it was caused by discomfort in the mouth and that it would end when his teeth were through. She said that his teeth now were through but there was no cessation of his dribbling. One doctor had said it was just a habit, and another had told her to make her child breathe through his nose. She described vividly how she was dreading the summer, when he would be too old for bibs though his cotton shirts would be soaked through in half an hour. She had also found that older children objected to being slobbered over by her baby.

I am full of sympathy for this mother, but at least I can set her mind at rest by assuring her that her baby is entirely normal and will come to no harm. I appreciate how distasteful it is to a mother to have her beautiful baby covered in dribble and regurgitated milk so that he not only looks bad but smells bad as well! Having seen hundreds of babies with this problem I have had hundreds of mothers making this point very clearly to me.

It is nothing to do with the teeth, nor is it the result of discomfort in the mouth. You only have to look at the baby as he wallows in the mess to realise how much he is enjoying himself. Mothers have so often emphasised to me the obvious pleasure their baby gets from the process and how he smiles and chuckles after he has brought up another nauseating dribble.

The doctor who said it was a habit is absolutely right, and a very enjoyable habit at that. All babies around the age of six months begin to derive enormous pleasure from their mouths. Once they have found it they want to cram into it everything they can get hold of. This may be enough to satisfy the majority of babies but some, like this one, wish for still more pleasure from their mouths. Such babies go on to the dribbling and regurgitating habit. The more their mothers dab their mouths the more they enjoy it and continue the practice since their mother is adding to their oral pleasure.

What can be done about it? The first thing is to be absolutely clear that it is doing the baby no harm, in fact it would be very unkind to try to stop him having such fun. The only reason for needing to do anything about it is the social consequence. No one wants to pick up the baby because he will spoil their clothes, and in any case his smell is revolting even though it doesn't worry him! Looked at in this way the problem becomes a laundry one rather than a health one. It should not matter how soaked his clothes become because there is no need to keep changing them – he won't catch cold from wearing a shirt he has made wet from dribbling.

The big thing is to avoid having your feelings of pride hurt by your messy, smelly baby. And don't keep dabbing his mouth because that tends to perpetuate the habit still more.

Concerning her child's breathing problem, you can't 'teach' a three-year-old to breathe through his nose but it would be an exceptional three-year-old who was breathing through his mouth. It is important not to confuse the child who keeps his mouth open (the open-mouth habit) with the child who is actually a mouth breather. These dribbling babies often retain for longer than usual the infantile pattern of keeping the mouth slightly open. You can test which way a child is breathing by putting a few threads of cotton wool in front of his mouth. See if they are blown down from his nose or out from his mouth.

There is one great compensation for the parents of dribbling babies. Almost all the ones I see, and I meet a very large number, are the gay, bright, extrovert type of child.

enough to eat 41.

All mothers are worried at some time that their children are not getting enough to eat. The strength of this fear comes from knowing that the young baby cannot look after himself and therefore could starve to death. Even if he didn't die there is the fear that he would become ill from lack of food. In a breast-feeding community these feelings are less intense, since mothers are not geared to seeing the amount of milk the baby has drunk, as is possible if he is fed by bottle. The breast-feeding mother is able more easily to judge that her baby has had enough milk on the basis that he seems satisfied, whereas the bottle-feeding mother is more likely to be concerned about quantities because she can see some milk left in the bottle. Her concern makes no allowance for the fact that no one wants the same amount at each feed and that the breast-fed baby varies in the amount he takes.

The major problem affecting the nutrition of children in Britain today is over-feeding. This could well be related to the swing to bottle-feeding and the emphasis on the quantity a baby should take, an approach which is continued when mixed feeding is started.

If a mother is not to lay emphasis on quantity how should she judge that her child has had enough food? For the baby, she should judge by the fact that he is thriving and content; that he sleeps peacefully between feeds with increasing periods of play as he grows older. Once old enough to crawl or run she should judge by his activity. A starved child is inactive. At the end of the last war I was involved in the repatriation of civilian prisoners of war from a camp in the middle of Java. When I entered the compound for the first time I could not think what was so strange in the children I was looking at. It was not malnutrition and the other horrors of war to which, sadly, one had become accustomed. It took a few seconds to realise that what was unusual was to be looking at hundreds of children who, though not asleep, were not moving. They were squatting, sitting or lying, nature thus ensuring that no food was being wasted in unnecessary energy. In reverse, therefore, the mother of an energetic child knows he is getting enough because the body, having taken all it needs for body building, has spare calories left over to keep him on the run.

An obsession with feeding is very likely to lead to battles over meals between the toddler and his mother. If a mother is very concerned that her young child should eat she will arouse his natural negativistic reactions so that he fights against her. Forcing a child to sit over his meals may cause him to vomit. The parents of such children sometimes express surprise that though the child vomits he does not seem to be upset by it – in fact he may seem better once he has vomited. If understood on the basis of the child's feelings it can be appreciated why such a child may feel better once he has vomited.

Because the young child wishes to please his mother a different reaction may result from her over-emphasis on food. He will try to eat to please her, but this only makes him feel unhappy because he does not want it. Such a child meets an extra turmoil when his mother threatens to remove the food he has not finished, since his desire to please her may take precedence, causing him to cry and say he will eat it up.

What, then, should the mother do to steer a middle pathway? She must avoid being concerned about the amount her child eats so that mealtime does not become an occasion for tension between them. Many children do not want a big breakfast before going off to school and hundreds of mothers could save themselves unnecessary anxiety because they feel their school child must have something warm inside him before he sets off – it is perfectly normal for a child not to want it.

The mother of the healthy child will always know he is having enough to eat simply because he is consistently energetic.

fat babies 42.

If you were to ask a mother to describe a 'bonny' baby she would probably give you a picture of a plump, cheerful infant. But why is fatness in babies associated with the concept of good health? At last we are aware that a fat adult is not in optimum health, but the same understanding for babies is uncommon. Mothers are far more concerned lest their babies are too thin rather than too fat. They look surprised and hurt when told their baby is too plump and it is exceptional for a mother to complain to her doctor that her baby weighs too much. Yet, in this country, obesity is the most common variety of malnutrition in babies.

What makes babies fat? In most cases it is starting cereal feeding too early and giving too much. One even hears of cereals being given while babies are still in the maternity ward. Doctors and nurses are sometimes as much to blame as mothers. It is difficult to discover the reasoning behind the giving of cereals to very young babies. I am sometimes told that it is needed to get the baby to go to sleep and that he is not satisfied with the ordinary amount of milk. But if a baby continues to cry despite an adequate milk intake there is probably some other reason for the crying. Many babies cry because their mothers are upset and distressed; babies are very accurate barometers of their mothers' feelings. Babies like to be cuddled and talked to at the end of a feed but mothers often make the mistake of putting them straight back to bed after the feed and then wonder why they cry.

By the time the baby is only a few weeks old he is beginning to take notice of his surroundings and to enjoy them. He spends less of his time asleep. Mothers should get away from the idea that the baby must be asleep all the time between meals, or be filled up with cereal if he dares to stay awake too long.

Does it matter if babies are too fat? The answer is a very emphatic yes. Fat babies make fat children and fat children make fat adults. The baby who has become used to too much food will crave for more when he is cut down, making a reduction in his excessive weight gain more difficult. Recent research has shown that when a growing child becomes too fat the cells in his body which contain the fat (adipose or fat cells) increase not only in size but also in number. This means that for the rest of his life he carries an extra number of fat cells all waiting to be filled up. No wonder it is so difficult to reduce the amount of fat once it has been laid down.

And there are other disadvantages in being too fat. It is fat babies who develop the tendency to wheeze. Wheezing in babies is now a common problem. Fat children become knock-kneed. The normal baby has slightly bowed legs and as he grows up into a toddler this change is reversed so that he develops a slight degree of knock knee. However, if he is too fat, what is a normal mild degree of knock knee becomes exaggerated and will persist until the extra weight is lost.

I am sometimes asked how soon you can diet a baby. The answer is: as soon as you find he is too fat. If the baby is on cereals they should be cut out altogether. If he is getting more than his share of milk it should be reduced. The normal amount of milk for a baby is 2½ ounces per pound of body weight per day. This must be based on his expected weight and not on his actual weight – a fat baby will otherwise go on being fed too much.

Protein rather than carbohydrate (as in cereal) is what the fat baby needs. Now that cheap food blenders are on the market it is an easy matter to make a mince of the meat that has been cooked for other members of the family, and fruit and vegetables can be similarly prepared.

The derivation of the word bonny is uncertain but it probably comes from the French word 'bon' meaning good. Fat babies are commonly 'good' in the sense that they are placid; but I would much prefer a baby to be active and curious about his surroundings, than to be sozzled into inactivity by too much food.

I have never accepted an invitation to judge a baby show, nor do I like the idea of them. However, if I did accept such an invitation I would want a year's notice so that it could be used to get the fat off the babies. One of the regulations I would make is that any baby weighing more than his expected normal would automatically be excluded!

more about fat babies 43.

The last piece on fat babies received so much support from mothers when it first appeared that I was encouraged to go into the question of obesity in more depth. There are still problems: one reader wrote, 'My health visitor is unalarmed at the possibility of my baby becoming overweight; she tells me "you cannot overfeed a baby".' How wrong she is! Fortunately, this attitude amongst health visitors is now exceptional and a recent correspondent in their journal, while complaining about those who recommend the early giving of cereals to young babies, said that in her area it was the paediatrician who was giving this advice. Obviously, no single professional body is free of blame.

Many readers, while accepting that cereals should not be given early, have asked for more detailed information as to when they can be given. The mother of a ten-week baby weighing 13 lbs asked when she could start cereals. These questions presuppose that cereals must be given some time, whereas I would avoid them altogether in a plump baby.

The difficulty in writing about infant feeding is that mothers want detailed instructions when it is far better that they should be taught general principles and then adapt an experimental approach to the feeding of their own baby – it is also more fun to experiment than to be rigid. Books on infant care, particularly of the Truby King era, used to give such detailed advice on quantities that mothers were frightened to move one step away from it.

By the time the child is a toddler most mothers are no longer requesting detailed information on the exact type and amount of food to be given, and when to give it. They are prepared to go by guidelines. I would like to achieve the same commonsense approach right from the start.

The trouble with cereals is that they are so easy to make up and to give; for years they have uncritically been regarded as the baby's first weaning food. A baby is much more likely to accept cereals than the savoury taste of meat. This means that a mother needs to be more subtle and persevering in the initial stages of giving meat foods. But there are many advantages to the baby if he is given a meat food in preference to cereal. Being protein it is a muscle builder rather than a maker of fat, like cereal. Getting used to the very different savoury taste of meat, though more difficult at first, means that he is likely to accept new tastes later on more easily than a baby fed milk and cereal only for the first months. Babies are conservative people who dislike change once they have become entrenched in their ways. It is believed that the taste buds on the tongue are not fully developed until the end of the first year, so the early introduction of new tastes slips them in before the baby is fully aware of the difference – an underhand physiological trick on the baby, but well worth while.

This is not to say that cereals should *never* be the first solid for the baby, but the decision to give cereals should be taken in the light of the individual baby's progress. Cereal is ideal for a small two-week baby who is crying from hunger, and obviously needs more calories than can be supplied from milk because he hasn't got enough room for all the ounces of milk this would require.

On the other hand, the baby who is large at birth and therefore likely to put on weight too rapidly should be given broth or meat in purée form as the first solid, rather than cereal. The same principles apply to the baby as to yourself. If you are fat it is to be hoped that you would not feed yourself bowls of porridge.

Broth can be given to a baby of two to three weeks if extra foods are needed by then. It can be home-made but, since this is time-consuming, most mothers will prefer the manufactured variety. In these early days, when only one or two spoonfuls are taken, much of a can would be wasted. This is where the meat and vegetable broths in powdered form come in so handy – they can be mixed with milk or water and you only need to mix the amount the baby wants.

When choosing baby foods in cans keep off those with added cereal. For example, buy plain beef rather than beef with cereal. Keep away from the syrupy desserts available from the manufacturers. It is much better to stew apples yourself, without sugar, and then put them through the blender if the baby is very young. Fresh orange juice or tomato juice is preferable to syrupy rose-hip juice.

The manufacturers' cans should be used as a convenience rather than a routine. Try and incorporate your own foods – meat, vegetable and fruit – into the baby's diet, liquidising them in the early weeks. Most household mincers have different-sized cutters, and the fine one produces chopped meat and vegetables which, when mixed into a paste with stock or gravy, gives a sufficiently smooth paste even for a very young baby. Meat left over from the adults' evening meal can safely be left covered overnight in the refrigerator and then put through the liquidiser or mincer in the morning and given to the baby. Children enjoy having the same foods as grown-ups, and at a very early age are aware if they are being given something different. Possibly this is one reason why they pick food off an adult's plate in preference to their own.

At the same time we should not project on to the baby our own preferences in relation to the timing of foods taken during the day. Just because we don't like minced meat or cauliflower for breakfast, there is no reason to think that the baby will share our prejudices.

Giving cereals early in life is a lazy habit. Because her baby takes it easily, a mother is gratifying her own mothering instincts in enjoying watching her baby feed, but she has really failed by not getting him to eat more suitable food. Before long, the increasing amounts of cereal demanded by the baby, together with a rusk or two, will have produced a fat baby. Much better to take the less easy path with meat and vegetables. It is very likely to be spat back at first but this doesn't matter. The baby who keeps spewing it back will probably change overnight and suddenly take it without difficulty provided his mother perseveres, at the same time avoiding a battle by an air of unconcern and a lack of fussing and coaxing. Try extra tricks such as giving the meat half way through the milk feed when the baby's initial hunger and thirst have been assuaged, and placing the food on the back of the tongue from where it is less easily spat back than if placed on the tip.

The early introduction of meat and vegetables not only has the advantage of early new tastes but there is the extra advantage of encouraging the baby to chew. Cereals don't need to be chewed, and the later introduction of lumpy foods will probably be resented by the baby.

Where does all this take us? As long as the baby who is on a milk-only diet – whether breast or bottle – is satisfied and not gaining weight excessively, the addition of solids can be left till about three months. If he is small and hungry he can be given cereal, but if he is large and hungry he should be given meat and vegetable. In judging his gain in weight, anything between 4 and 8 ounces a week is probably all right. Obviously, the baby's actual weight will depend on the figure he started with at birth. But scales are not necessary to judge whether he is overweight – if he looks fat then adjust his foods accordingly. At a very early stage, four to six months, let him dip his fingers into the food and start to feed himself. It will be messy and some will go in his hair but he will enjoy the experience. In some ways it is a good idea for food to go into his hair because it doesn't make him fat like food going into his mouth.

Also at an early stage let him experiment with a spoon, even though this too will be messy. His mother should have a second spoon for greater accuracy in getting food into his mouth.

Above all, adopt an experimental approach to the feeding of babies, and let the baby take part in the experiment as well.

going to pot 44.

While some mothers are obsessive about the amount of food their children eat, others are similarly concerned about a regular daily bowel action from their children. This anxiety is not confined to mothers – a desperately worried father once said to me, 'my child must have his bowels open every day, otherwise he'll die'! This mechanical approach to the body's natural functions fails to appreciate that left alone the body works perfectly well. I have never heard of a dog owner being concerned about her pet's bowels and the dog comes to no harm. Why can't we adopt the same attitude to children's bowels?

Concern about bowels appears to have been particularly emphasised in the last century and is one of the most catching of habits, being passed from parent to child through the generations. It is likely to have started with excessive concern over early pot-training in the belief that a child trained early to use the pot will become 'clean' at an early age. The very use of the word 'clean' to describe the acquisition of this art suggests that the other babies are dirty. Bound up with this is the belief that early training will ensure a regular daily habit.

Mothers are competitive over the skills attained by their children so that to become 'clean' at an early age is regarded as a praiseworthy achievement. Unfortunately, early pot-training disregards the normal developmental processes of the child. Any child, whether bright or dull, can be trained from an early age to have his bowels open when sat on a pot. This is a 'conditioned reflex' and in this case the touch of the pot on the skin of the bottom triggers the reflex mechanism causing the bowels to function. No willpower is involved in the reflex so that all goes well for the first months before voluntary willpower develops towards the end of the first year.

Once this willpower has developed, the child is likely to assert himself so that he fights against the reflex. Not only does he hold on to his bowels to prevent their opening but he also may refuse to sit on the pot, particularly if his mother tries to make him do so. If a mother fails to recognise the reason for his behaviour she is likely to force him to sit on the pot, causing him to scream and to refuse to have his bowels open for increasingly long periods.

Pot-training, therefore, though useful in saving laundry, carries snags and the wise mother will avoid attempting it. If she does go in for pot-training she must recognise the signals just described which indicate a reaction from the child. To deal with this the child should be put back into nappies, no attempt being made to reintroduce the pot for two or three months. By this means she is removing the circumstances causing her child to do battle with her, so preventing bowel actions from becoming an area of conflict between herself and her child.

Parents who are themselves bowel-conscious need to understand that their concern may make them think of their child as a bowel which must be made to open at the times they believe to be right. In the same way that excessive concern over a child's meals leads to food refusal, so excessive concern over bowels leads to bowel refusal, that is, constipation. This negativistic reaction is part of the normal developing behaviour pattern of the child which in the circumstances cited has been caused to become excessive.

Is constipation harmful? Judging by the list of symptoms put out by the makers of laxative pills one would think so, but the majority of these symptoms are imaginary, being indulged in only by bowel-conscious individuals. The major symptom of constipation in childhood is possibly the least expected – diarrhoea. This is due to overflow caused by over-filling of the rectum and stretching of the anus. Abdominal pain is minimal in most cases, though the straining caused by a child subconsciously trying to hold on to his bowels to prevent their opening may be misinterpreted as a painful bowel action.

Tiredness, insomnia, bad breath and similar symptoms, although strongly promoted by the laxative manufacturers, are unrealistic indications of constipation and are adult-inspired.

The average householder does not make a daily check of his drains to see if his house is in good shape. We should avoid the mistake of trying to assess the health of a child by his daily bowel action.

45. bed-wetting

There can be few parents who have not at some time been worried about their child wetting his bed, but the number of adults who still wet the bed is not great. Parents can therefore be comforted by the fact that their child is almost certain to lose the habit during childhood.

Much of the problem results from parents trying too hard, at an early age, to make their child dry. A normal child may still be wetting the bed up to the age of four even though many children gain control earlier. This means that if the child is otherwise normal parents of bed-wetters should wait until he is four before feeling they must consult their doctor. The doctor will always check that the child is physically normal, which is usually the case. Physical causes are more likely if the child is always damp, if he dribbles urine instead of passing a normal stream or if he suddenly starts to wet after a long period of being dry. All these are reasons for consulting the doctor early.

Quite often one of the parents was late in gaining control, a fact which supports the belief that bed-wetting is due to a delay in the normal development of bladder control and that this may be inherited.

There is much that can be done to help a child become dry. Most children gain control during the day first because it is easier when they are awake. But parents can help the night problem by shortening the period their child is expected to stay dry. Bedtime can come later, provided the child is not being a nuisance to his parents. He should pass water just before getting into bed and his mother or father should lift him just before they go to bed themselves. If he is ever wet at that time an extra lift should be carried out some time between the child's and his parents' bedtime. In this way, parents can ensure the child is always dry when they go to bed.

The method of lifting is important. The child should use a pot beside his bed rather than being sent down a cold corridor to the lavatory, to which he is likely to object strongly. There is no need to wake him up; all that is required is that the bladder should be emptied. Many children use the pot without seeming to wake up and that is perfectly all right.

The last lift should be undertaken by whichever parent gets up first in the morning, even before he uses the lavatory himself. This prevents the child being disturbed by the household noises so that in a half-wakeful state he wets his bed.

There should be no restriction of fluids in the evening. This causes distress and is quite unnecessary. On no account should a child be scolded or punished for wetting his bed since this only prolongs the problem. The whole approach is one of praise for dry nights and no comment on the wet ones.

A prize for each dry night is much more effective than the promise of a bicycle when dry which may be months away. A suitable prize is a penny; this should be placed by his mother beside her child's money box, away from his bed, when she tucks him up at night. This method ensures that the child's last waking thoughts are of how he can earn his prize. When he gets up in the morning, and provided he is dry, he puts the prize in the money box. If wet, his mother, without comment, removes the prize and resets the trap the next evening. Interestingly enough, I have never found a child to cheat and put the money in the box when he has actually wet the bed.

Boys wet the bed more often than girls because

they have possibly been supplied with smaller bladders. Their bladders can be stretched and the stimulus to empty the bladder can be reduced by what is termed 'day-clock training'. During the day his mother, using an alarm clock, gets her child to go for increasing lengths of time without passing urine. She might start at two-hourly intervals and gradually increase to four or five hours.

Enthusiasm is the keynote for success, and once a mother has seen her child can be dry throughout one night she knows that his kidneys cannot be at fault – something which may have been worrying her. An outside source of praise is helpful, and the doctor can assist if he lets the child bring him a calendar on which he has ringed his dry nights. Alternatively, the child may enjoy bringing the contents of his money box to show him.

The electric buzzer is often useful with older children but drugs are not much help, and are certainly poor substitutes for the doctor who is prepared to spend time and by own enthusiasm, help the child to a lasting cure.

46. the bedtime battleground

The main reason for putting a child to bed is to give his parents a rest. Once parents have accepted the truth of this very human reason for wanting their children to go to bed they can begin to get away from the old-fashioned, though still widely held, belief that a specific number of hours of sleep is required for each child, depending on his age. Unfortunately, it is still possible for mothers to read articles which list the number of hours of sleep required for each year of a child's life. This mechanical approach to sleep takes no account of the enormous individual variations in the sleep requirements of children as well of adults.

Parents who believe that their child must go to sleep for the sake of his health soon convey their anxiety to the child, who is liable to stay awake worrying because he can't get to sleep. The child not brought up with this ritual will be able to drop off to sleep as soon as he needs it, even if he hasn't been put to bed. British parents holidaying in France are often critical of French parents bringing their young children to the restaurant in the evening instead of leaving them at home in bed. But we should also consider the possibility that it is much nicer for the child to stay with the family rather than be left with a babysitter, and this experience of going out as a family is good for him. If he wants to go to sleep he can easily do so at the table, as in fact he will often do. Parents can enjoy their children more if they can get away from the rigid ideas connected to bedtime.

The brighter the infant, the more is he likely to wake up early in the morning and want to play. This is liable to be intensely irritating to his parents, whose sleep requirements are probably greater than his. However, they can get some comfort from knowing that he is possibly brighter than the average child and that far from harming him this extra play is of benefit. Since a child learns through play it is as though he is opting for overtime to do more work. The way the parents should handle this problem is not to tell the child to go to sleep, which is useless, but to provide him with suitable toys in the hope that he will amuse himself so that they can go back to sleep or better still not be woken at all even when he wakes.

Bedtime should be fun for children and parents rather than becoming a battleground. Children who are enjoying a game should be given a warning that it is nearly time for bed rather than abruptly being told to stop in the middle of the game. The young child should be given an opportunity to 'unwind' from his exciting game – ideally by a story on his mother's knee. This is one of the golden moments in the day when parent and child can get closer – it should not be lost in the hurry to get the child to sleep.

The older child should be allowed to read in bed, and if the decision to turn his light off is left to him a battle is avoided and the child's reading encouraged. Similarly, he should know that he can read in the early morning if he wants to.

What else can be done to help parents get the rest they need? From a very early age the baby should have a 'room' of his own rather than sleeping in the parents' room. This can be achieved even if there is only one bedroom, either by moving the baby into the living room when the parents go to bed or by having his cot on a landing. Habit, too, plays a large part in encouraging sleep, and the child who knows he cannot call his mother back is much more likely to go straight off to sleep than one who can get her back every time he calls.

Right from the start, parents should accustom their babies to sleeping through noise. Those who adopt the attitude of 'Hush! You'll wake the baby' saddle themselves with a baby who wakes at the slightest noise. On the other hand, the baby who starts off by sleeping despite the television and other noises will be given an asset for life.

The longer the child's rest in the day the less likely will he be to sleep at night. The sooner this rest period can be dropped the easier the nights will be.

These views are far removed from the absurd remarks which parents still hear, such as 'His brain will tire if he doesn't get enough sleep'. It will be obvious from what has been said that sedatives are not a form of treatment for children who cannot get to sleep.

47. convulsions

Convulsions – or fits as they are often called – are always alarming but fortunately the most common type in children – febrile convulsions – is the least serious. A high fever in any young child may set off a convulsion, the usual cause of the fever being a throat or an ear infection. Fits most usually occur between the ages of one and three years. Fever is rarely the cause of a convulsion in the first year of life; children who get them are toddlers rather than babies. Quite often, another member of the family in the same or a previous generation will have had similar attacks when young.

The best way to prevent the fit is to bring down the child's temperature. A child who is feverish needs to be cooled, just as an adult does when he feels hot. As a first step all bedding and clothes should be removed, but if this is insufficient to make him cool, and particularly if the temperature is above 103°F, the young child should be tepid-sponged. To do this he lies naked on a mackintosh on the bed or in an empty bath. Tepid water is then sponged over him and allowed to dry by evaporation; this causes the temperature of the skin to fall. Tepid sponging should be continued until the temperature falls to 102°F. Cold water is not used as it causes the blood vessels in the skin to contract so the result is much less effective.

In addition to tepid sponging the child can be given one junior aspirin tablet or half an adult aspirin to help bring down the temperature. It will be the doctor's task to diagnose the cause of the fever and to decide whether antibiotic treatment is required.

Febrile convulsions are unnecessarily common due to the lingering and very mistaken belief that a child who is feverish must be kept warm. How often one is called to a feverish child, only to find him with a jersey over his pyjamas, blankets over his sheets and the windows closed. The look of horror on his mother's face when you open the windows and remove the extra clothing indicates the strength of this belief, which dates back to Victorian times.

What should be done if, despite these precautions, the child starts to convulse? The first thing is not to panic; stay with the child, don't rush out for help and leave him alone. A convulsion by itself never kills a child but it is dangerous if, while unconscious from the fit, he vomits and then inhales some of the vomit into his lungs. Tragedies have happened when a mother has rushed out of the house to call a neighbour, leaving the child alone. Moreover, a child will be terrified if he finds himself alone on coming round from the convulsion. The convulsion will only last a minute or two. During this time he is best left on the bed, his mother beside it to prevent him falling off. No attempt should be made to force open his mouth in order to make him breathe or to stop him biting his tongue. He will breathe when the stiffness has left him and children seldom bite the tongue. Much more damage will be done by trying to force open his mouth.

Doctors still debate about whether giving anticonvulsant drugs, such as phenobarbitone, between attacks reduces the liability to febrile convulsions. Present evidence is that this is ineffective, so that fewer and fewer doctors are prescribing these drugs for this type of convulsion. The measures to bring down the temperature are certainly far more effective. Constipation and worms are not causes of convulsions.

Parents will wish to know whether the child who has a febrile convulsion is going to be an 'epileptic'. The chances of this are very small, since epilepsy rarely starts in young children. A useful indication of future progress will come from the pattern of febrile convulsions in other members of the family if these have occurred, as the pattern of this disorder in families remains strikingly similar. The doctor will be helped to some extent by the result of an electroencephalogram – a tracing on paper of the electrical waves from the brain. In most children with febrile convulsions the electroencephalogram is normal.

Epileptic convulsions more often occur out of the blue rather than being caused by a fever. The muscular exercise involved in the convulsion may cause the temperature to rise after the fit has started, but this is a different matter, although it sometimes leads to confusion.

The outlook for children with epilepsy is very different today from what it used to be. This change is due partly to a wider variety of medicines to combat the problem and partly to a different attitude to epilepsy among doctors and the general public. If, after a suitable trial period, a child fails to respond to one medicine he will be tried on another, either alone or in combination with the first. Today's approach to treatment is that the doctor should go on making adjustments in the medicines until he stops the convulsions altogether. He will then keep the child on the effective medicine for a long period, usually three years from the last convulsion, before slowly withdrawing it.

No longer is a child labelled as 'an epileptic'. As far as possible he should be treated as a normal child and almost always he should attend an ordinary rather than a special school. Restrictions should be minimal; he should not bicycle unless accompanied by an adult but swimming is possible, provided an adult agrees to keep an eye on him alone the whole time he is in the water.

It is now realised that the altered personality ascribed to 'epileptics' in the past largely resulted from their being herded away together and ostracised by society.

breath-holding attacks 48. and faints

Apart from convulsions there are two other types of attack in children which may lead to loss of consciousness. These occur at either end of childhood, breath-holding attacks being confined to the toddler age group while fainting attacks are a problem for the older child.

The toddler who develops breath-holding attacks is always bright and strong-willed. He is easily frustrated and his temper is such that he reacts to frustration by holding his breath. The attack is brought on by anything which annoys him – for example, if a toy he is playing with is taken from him. Sometimes an attack is precipitated by his falling down and hurting himself, as though he is furious with the ground for coming up and hitting him. Like any actor these children must have an audience for their performance, and do not have attacks when they are on their own. In fact, they seldom have an attack unless one of their parents is present.

The usual sequence is that after the precipitating event the child takes a big breath as though he is about to produce the biggest-ever cry. However, instead of emitting any noise he holds his breath, going red and then blue in the face. Less often the child may cry for a short time and then hold his breath. If the breath is held for long enough, lack of oxygen causes loss of consciousness followed by an actual convulsion.

Parents of such children find themselves in a cleft stick resulting from their fear of doing anything which may precipitate their child's temper and subsequent breath-holding attacks, which are very alarming. However, they and the child soon become aware of the consequences of this policy so that the child becomes increasingly unmanageable. If some means can be found to stop short the attack, equilibrium between child and parents can be restored.

Most parents will find that slapping the child to make him breathe or throwing cold water at him makes little difference. A useful trick which often works is to insert the index finger into the child's mouth and hook it over the back of the tongue. Pulling the finger forward while in that position pulls the tongue forward and causes a reflex so that the child takes a breath. Once one breath has been taken the attack always stops.

It is some relief to parents faced with these alarming attacks to know that the child will always come round. He will also always lose the habit as he grows older although his strong determination is likely to continue to show itself in other ways.

Fainting attacks occur mainly in the second half of childhood, particularly when the child is growing fast just before adolescence. He feels faint, thinks he is going to be sick and looks a deathly white colour. No convulsive movements occur and he does not wet himself.

The cause of the attack is insufficient blood supply to the brain. The immediate treatment is to loosen any tight clothing round his neck and to put his head between his knees in order to increase the amount of blood reaching the brain. Plenty of fresh air should be allowed to reach the child. A drink of water on recovery is usually welcome.

These attacks occur only when the child is standing, and by far the most frequent occasion for them is at 'school assembly' in the morning. It would be difficult to arrange better conditions for the production of faints. The children have rushed to school early in the morning after a hurried breakfast and then have to stand together in a crowded and stuffy hall. Prevention of the attacks lies in permitting the children to sit down during assembly. To those headmasters and headmistresses who say that there are insufficient chairs to permit all the children to sit, the answer is to insist that they are allowed to sit on the floor.

The problem at school assembly is not simply the attacks themselves but also the effects on other children. For every child who faints there are many more who are frightened in case they too will do so.

Irritating habits 49.

How should you deal with those irritating habits acquired by babies and children, such as head banging, rocking, blinking and nail biting? Can you accept the advice you are bound to get from someone that you need not worry since your child is sure to grow out of the habit?

FORMING HABITS

The answer is that you cannot sit back and leave nature to take its course. There is a reason for each habit and your child will be happier if you can discover this, even though the habit itself will probably disappear on its own with time.

Head banging and rocking are habits acquired by some babies around the age of nine to 12 months. Such habits should be taken seriously because they indicate that something has gone wrong with the mother-child relationship. In the early months a baby is comforted by being rocked in his mother's arms, but after a few months he grows out of the need for this particular form of physical comfort. This is partly, perhaps, because he is more aware of his mother as a person who radiates comfort, and partly because his natural curiosity and growing awareness of all the exciting things going on around him remove the need for such monotonous physical comfort.

A baby who begins to rock and to bang his head is having to do this to comfort himself. What has happened to cause his natural development to be diverted into these repetitive habits which waste his time and reduce his natural opportunity for learning? Certainly there must be an element of insecurity and also of boredom. Perhaps the baby is being left on his own too long. He needs the stimulus of being near his mother so that he can watch what she is doing. Even if his mother is busy in the kitchen, the baby can be propped up in his special chair to watch her.

The mother of such a baby should spend as much time as possible with him and should try to attract his attention by some interesting game with him. If this fails, she should satisfy his need for extra comfort by cuddling rather than leaving him to find it for himself by rocking.

Blinking, sniffing, shoulder shrugging and face twitching are habits which affect older children. The habit may have started with a purpose, for example tossing the head back to get a lock of hair out of the eyes, but continues when the original cause no longer exists. These are commonly called nervous habits and it is true that they usually reflect inward anxiety.

The treatment of such a habit involves getting to the bottom of the child's emotional problem and steadfastly avoiding telling him to stop the movement; this only makes the habit worse and the child more embarrassed.

Nail biting often runs in families so that I commonly find I am faced with a child and his mother both with bitten nails. It often seems to reflect a failure to control inward tension. Throughout most of the day the child can control this habit because he knows it meets with disapproval; during periods of excitement, however, such as a television programme, his control is lost, his subconscious anxiety comes to the surface and he finds he has bitten his nails. Perhaps a string of 'worry beads' to play with, such as those commonly carried by Arab men, would save the nails.

A useful trick to help girls who bite their nails is to give them their own bottle of colourless nail varnish. A girl is likely to be proud that she is allowed nail varnish and will want to show it off, so she will let her nails grow. It is essential to enlist the co-operation of her teacher so that she knows this is 'medical' nail varnish. Painting the nails with bitter substances, or other forms of punishment, only makes a child defiant so that it has the opposite of the desired effect.

PART FIVE
PARENTAL APPROACHES

50. management not punishment

It is in this field that an understanding of child development is essential. For the first year of his life the child cannot be expected to discriminate between what is right and what is wrong. Normal parents will therefore not punish their child for crying, wetting or making a mess. But they should know that it is normal for them sometimes to feel cross with the baby even though they know he couldn't help doing whatever it was that upset them. If a mother has tried all she can to stop her baby crying but he still persists, then she should go away and make herself a cup of tea rather than allowing herself to become even more distraught by his crying.

During his second year a child begins to develop his own willpower, and finds that he can manipulate his parents by what he does. It is during the toddler age that the child shows negativistic behaviour, and may refuse his food or to sit on the pot. He may refuse to speak the words his parents try to get him to say or refuse to walk, being perfectly happy with his crawling. It would be absurd to punish him for any of these failures, while attempts to persuade him by bribes and other measures to undertake these tasks would only increase his awareness of his new-found power over his parents.

Parents should not expect too much of their young children so that their bad behaviour disappoints them. They should also avoid making too many rules, thereby forcing themselves to take action against their young children over trivial issues.

In considering how to discipline a child it should be clearly understood that intuitively a child wishes to behave well because he does not want to lose his parents' favour. Wise management of the child is therefore much better than punishment. Time should be spent in considering why the child was 'naughty' since a child sometimes behaves in this way when he needs to attract his mother's attention.

Stealing is a useful example to consider in relation both to age and to underlying causes. If a baby takes a toy from another child he is stealing, but no one would consider punishing him for this: its significance therefore increases with the age of the child. But a child who knows it is wrong to steal may do so in such a way that he is sure to be found out because he is using this as a method of crying for help; it is essential for parents to recognise such a cry from an emotionally disturbed child. Another child may steal because he has no pocket money or few, if any, personal possessions – everyone want to own something. A child who feels lonely and unloved may steal in order to be able to give away the stolen object; it is as though he is trying to buy love.

Physical punishment produces such complicated reactions in the child, as well as in the parents, that it is best avoided if possible. The child is likely to feel angry with the parent who inflicted the punishment and his feelings of anger may be so intense that he is frightened by them. The parent, on the other hand, is likely to feel guilty, especially if he has made the bad error of beating the child when he was feeling angry.

Children need to be helped to understand that angry feelings are normal, whereas parents must understand that when a child says he hates them, this is, in fact, what he feels at that moment but it does not mean he has stopped loving them as well. It is these mixed feelings of love and hate which are so bewildering to a child. The child may even say that he wished his mother were dead and then be frightened lest he might cause her death or at least make her unwell. For this reason a mother must never say that her child has made her ill, because he needs to learn that his anger is not as destructive as he feels. He also needs to learn that his parents' love for him continues despite the temporary anger he felt against them.

Another reason against physical punishment is that children should not learn aggressive behaviour from their parents; it should be left to children to learn it from each other.

Advocating fewer rules does not mean doing without them altogether. Children like to have some rules so that they know where they stand. The spoiled child who has always got his own way at home finds the outside world unnecessarily harsh when he reaches it. The toddler whose temper tantrum prevents him from being reasoned with is best left on his own to get over it. As long as his mother is there he is likely to continue with the act, whereas if she walks into the next room but leaves the door open he will probably stop his performance; no actor likes performing to an empty house!

Parents should agree on the standards of behaviour they require from their children. A child who is spoilt by one parent and thrashed by the other will soon drive a wedge between them. In discussing their differences, parents should understand that they are being influenced by their own upbringing. The parent brought up strictly as a child may either repeat the process with his own children or react the other way and refuse to take part in their discipline.

If punishment is necessary, it should be immediate rather than stored up, for example until the child's father comes home. The removal of a privilege, such as watching television or the after-meal sweet, is preferable to physical methods of punishment. On no account should the child be sent to bed as a punishment. Bed is a child's castle where he feels snug at night – it cannot serve the dual function of prison cell during the daytime.

Whatever punishment is used a child *must* understand that it is given because his parents dislike his behaviour and not because they dislike him.

talking by listening 51.

Children learn to speak by first listening to the sounds made by others. They must learn to hear before they can learn to speak. This explains why deafness is such an important cause of delay in the development of speech and why it must be recognised and treated by hearing aids at the earliest moment.

If a mother suspects that her child is not hearing properly she must have his hearing tested by an expert. The mother must not be fobbed off by some ignorant individual who tells her that it is too early for her child to be tested and that she should bring him back when he is older. Priceless weeks and months have been lost in this way. A baby's hearing can be tested when he is a few weeks old so that a diagnosis of defective hearing should certainly be made by the time he is six months old. Today, health visitors as well as doctors are trained to undertake routine hearing tests on all young babies.

Since hearing comes before speech a mother must ensure that her young baby often hears her speaking to him. This is also important for the development of a close bond between them. It has been wisely said that speech is learnt at knee level, meaning that it is when the baby is on his mother's knee that he learns to speak. Some mothers don't find it easy to talk to their young babies and I remember one mother who said it was something you did to dogs but that she would feel stupid if she did it to her baby.

A mother's role in the early days of her baby's speech development is to encourage his babbling by copying his sounds but picking out and re- peating those which are meaningful. It is in this way that he comes to say 'Mum-Mum' and 'Dad-Dad' in the early days, since these are the sounds which she encourages and reinforces, at the same time as she gives them meaning to her child. Her encouragement and obvious delight at his success give both of them the stimulus for new words to be learnt and, by attaching meaningful sounds to the objects to which they refer, her child builds up his vocabulary of words for the objects he sees in his daily life.

It will be obvious, therefore, that the mother who is silent with her child places him at a disadvantage in relation to the development of speech. Similarly, parents who are non-stop talkers among themselves are sending sounds over the head of their baby instead of encouraging his own sounds on a personal basis. They are also denying him the opportunity to speak so that he misses the practice which is so essential for the development of speech.

A balance is required between the silent mother on the one hand, and on the other the mother who is excessively concerned to make her child speak early. The mother who tries over-hard to make her child say the words she wants runs into the same problems as the mother who tries too hard to make her child eat the foods she wants him to. In the case of food his negativistic reactions may be evoked so that he will refuse his food; in the same way a mother's concern can lead to speech refusal. In the case of speech refusal the child may get along happily with grunt language, having achieved a delicious situation where his mother has become a slave to his grunts which she interprets with ease, running at his beck and call to undertake his grunt commands. The more the parents try to force him to say words the more entrenched does he become behind his grunt barrier. Such parents can be assured that their child is bright if he has achieved a language all of his own, and that when he mixes with other children who do not know his grunt language and are certainly not going to bother to learn it he will start to speak normally.

Possibly it is the fear that mental handicap is the cause of a child's delayed speech which drives parents to try to make their child speak. Mental handicap is a major cause of slow speech development, but such children show other evidence of backwardness as well.

pets or pet aversions 52.

Should you buy your child a pet? I believe it is an excellent thing for children to own a pet. The young child, like every normal being, wants to love and to be loved. Looking after a pet gives him an extra opportunity to express this natural desire to care for someone else.

Children living on farms have little difficulty in understanding the facts of life – mating, birth and death. A pet gives parents innumerable opportunities for helping their child to understand these basic facts.

In addition to providing opportunities for this factual knowledge a pet is someone on whom a child can lavish all his natural caring instincts. Time spent on feeding a kitten or a puppy is worth hours of explanation about his own behaviour at mealtimes and why his mother is so keen for him to eat up the food she has provided for him. Moreover, the fact that a mother can accept a messy puppy or kitten may help her to accept the messes made by her own child.

The young child is busy trying to learn to control his feelings. To help him do this he needs to control someone or something. The pet fits naturally into this role and the pet's reactions to some of the controlling measures applied by a child help the child to understand that no one likes to be controlled all the time, although some controls are essential. The nip or scratch resulting from pulling the pet's tail can be a salutary reminder to the child of the need to accept an individual's wishes and what can happen when feelings are hurt. From such experiences a child comes to understand problems involving feelings, whereas he is less able to accept these explanations from his mother.

A pet will deepen a child's emotions by

involving them more. This will be greatest when his pet dies. However, because this possibility exists do not make the mistake of trying to shelter him from it by not giving him a pet. For the same reason, do not immediately rush out to the pet shop to replace his dead pet. Give him time to mourn his loss since this is an essential human need to help recovery from the shock and distress of bereavement. If you were immediately to replace his dead pet you would also be making him think that the loss of any loved one could immediately be neutralised in this way. This would not help his understanding of life and death which a pet can do so much to foster.

Inevitably, a pet will mean more work for parents but the gain is well worth it. However, despite a child's promise that he will do all the looking after, parents must accept before they go off to the pet shop that they will have to undertake much of this extra work. The child's promise means that he intends to do all the work, but inevitably he won't. It is essential to accept the limitations of his age so that when some other activity makes him forget his pet's mealtime, he is not always called back to do his duty. Parents should be prepared to help without always scolding their child for forgetting. A child cannot be expected to learn all the responsibilities of a mother as soon as he owns a pet. Remember always that the pet is providing a superb learning experience for your child, whatever its drawbacks for you.

The ultimate responsibility for a pet's survival must remain with the parents. A child should not be given an unnecessary lesson in death, associated with recriminations on both sides that neither of you looked after the pet properly.

The choice of pet must be left to personal taste and the facilities available. I hope also that your children will be in contact with pets at school and in hospital. At school, rabbits and hamsters are more suitable than dogs and cats. In hospital, it is possible to have warm-blooded animals as well as the cold-blooded fish. In my wards we have for some time had guinea pigs, who have become important members of staff in the help they provide for the children. Visitors often ask about the risk of infection but this is greatly exaggerated.

Of course, the diseases caused by pets are important but they can be treated. The most frequent are skin disorders caused by fleas and mites from dogs and cats. These may result from direct infection of the skin but can very often be due to an allergic reaction to the body of the flea – even, therefore, to dead fleas in upholstery.

To treat these disorders successfully it is essential first to make a correct diagnosis. Unfortunately, people are very touchy when asked about the possibility of fleas in their house; doctors therefore have to proceed with great caution in the way they put their questions. Fleas are so closely associated in people's minds with dirt and filth that it is as though a slur has been cast on the household in even querying the possibility of fleas.

Worms can be passed from dogs to children, but although most puppies have worms I do not think the frequency with which this transference occurs is all that great. In any case, the worms are relatively harmless and can easily be treated with the medicines now available.

The really serious illnesses like rabies are prevented by our strict quarantine rules. Another serious infection, psittacosis, is caught from birds such as budgerigars and parrots; it can be avoided by purchasing such pets only after they have been immunised. It is well worth paying the extra money and I would advise you to patronise those pet shops which provide this sort of extra care and skill for the pets they sell.

games children play 53.

The young child has very intense likes and dislikes. Some of these, particularly in the toddler age group, lead to forms of behaviour which need to be understood by parents in order to help the child. These are not ordinary games in the sense that the child consciously plans to play them; rather are they 'games' which originate in the subsconscious part of the child's mind. The child does not plan his mode of behaviour in these 'games', nor does he understand why he is behaving in the way he does. However, it is essential that parents should understand what is going on in order to guide their child out of the conflict which has produced this train of reactions.

Negativism is a good example of such behaviour. It appears in various forms, depending on which area of the child's life the parent is trying to mould most strongly to conform with his or her own beliefs of what is good for the child.

A simple example of this is excessive concern over eating, which usually happens during the second half of the child's first year. Up till then the baby has probably taken the breast or bottle without much difficulty, but now his awakening ability to manipulate his mother can take charge if she becomes over-concerned about regimenting him. This may show itself in a refusal to switch from bottle to spoon-feeding or in keeping his mouth tightly closed and turning the head away when his mother approaches with food. If she goes on trying to force him to eat, the child may vomit, sometimes sticking his fingers down his throat to achieve it.

The answer is to understand the child's behaviour in terms of what has evoked it and to switch that off. The baby who makes the change from bottle to solids by being allowed to stick his fingers in the food and carry it to his mouth is unlikely to run into this difficulty. He will accept spoon-feeding with ease because his mother is not being intense about it and very soon he will be able to wield the spoon himself with accuracy.

Speech is another area in which parental concern for the child to speak words can evoke a negativistic reaction, and I have discussed this in the piece 'Talking by listening' on page 137.

Excessive attempts to make a child walk may result in his remaining longer in the crawling stage. Excessive concern to make a child go to sleep cause him to react by trying to keep awake. His parents are likely to interpret his irritability as due to lack of sleep instead of realising that it is the result of the turmoil they have produced.

Concern over pot-training is likely to make a child refuse to have his bowels open. The efforts to prevent the passage of a stool are likely to be misinterpreted by the parents as straining to have his bowels open. If the parents are excessively bowel conscious, so that a part of every day is spent in trying to get the child to have his bowels open, it is not uncommon for the child to hold on for up to two to three weeks. The parents of such a child are likely to tell the doctor that for the few days before he has his bowels open, the child is very irritable and is seen to be straining to open his bowels. In actual fact, the child is straining to hold on. If he were straining to have his bowels open he would squat in an appropriate position but instead of this he commonly stands up stiffly and often clenches his fists. One such child would push back the stool when it was half way out. His parents misinterpreted this as a sign of excessive pain on defecation. If this had been the case he would not have pushed it back so that he had to go through the 'painful' process again. Examination showed that he could pass a motion without physical pain.

Babies who cry excessively are often described as being bad-tempered instead of it being realised that their crying is a reaction to their distressed feelings. These feelings have usually come from the mother, who is crying inwardly if not visibly.

I do not believe that there is such a thing as a lazy child. Children behave in a way which adults interpret as laziness when really it is the result of a conflict between child and parents or child and school which has evoked a refusal reaction.

Even the youngest child is sensitive to his parents' feelings, and parents have to walk a tightrope. If they fall one way it is because over-involvement and over-protection have evoked a negativistic reaction. On the other hand, coldness and aloofness, particularly on the part of the mother, leads to lack of mothering and its problems. The young child who lacks proper mothering fails to thrive physically as well as emotionally, and lack of mothering in childhood leads to an inability of the child, when adult, to mother her own children.

54. helping with acne

It seems harsh that many children, in addition to facing the turbulent feelings which come to the surface during adolescence, should also have to cope with the disfigurement caused by acne.

Acne produces blackheads and those ugly red and white spots on the face which are the bane of so many adolescents. The same spots also turn up on the back of the neck and over the shoulders, but it is the ones on the face which really cause embarrassment.

Although girls as well as boys get acne it is worse in boys. The trouble comes from the sebaceous glands, whose job it is to produce the natural grease required by the skin. At puberty, these glands grow larger and produce more grease as a result of the hormone changes going on in the body. Those people with particularly greasy skins are the most likely to develop acne. There are more sebaceous glands on the face than elsewhere and this is the reason why the face is especially affected.

Sebaceous glands are sited alongside the root of the hair. The channel into which the grease (sebum) flows from these glands opens into the hair follicle which houses the root of the hair. Although the sebaceous glands get bigger at puberty there is no corresponding increase in the size of their channels or of the hair follicles. In people with acne this skin pore becomes blocked with horny material. This horny plug is the 'blackhead'; it is black from melanin, the colouring matter of the skin and hair, and not from ingrained dirt as used to be thought.

It is characteristic of all the body channels that, to remain healthy, they must be free of obstruction. Blockage of any body channel leads to inflammation. By blocking the pore the blackhead causes inflammation of the skin. This inflammation is not bacterial but chemical, being due to excess fatty acids derived from the sebum; it produces a raised red spot like a small boil. Pus can be formed inside this boil causing a pustule which is a yellowish-white spot on the skin. If the inflammation in the skin has been sufficiently deep, permanent scarring results.

Individuals who have the excessive greasiness of the skin which leads to acne are also likely to have scurf. This scurf exaggerates the tendency to acne.

By understanding why acne occurs, treatment is easier. The prime object of treatment is to prevent the formation of blackheads. It also aims to get rid of those which have developed before they produce the inflammation which causes the spots. The chief way to cut down the formation of blackheads is to wash the face vigorously as often as possible with hot water and soap, even using a scrubbing brush. The water should be as hot as can be tolerated; any soap will do. Hot water opens up the pores in the skin, thereby encouraging the flow of sebum. Soap washes away this sebum.

Scurf must be kept down by frequent shampooing with any of the medicated shampoos available. This should be done at least twice a week, but even every night if this is necessary to keep down the scurf.

Now that the chemical cause of acne from excess fatty acids is better understood, it is realised that the role of secondary infection has been exaggerated. In the past, sufferers from acne were warned of the risks of infection if blackheads were squeezed. Today, some dermatologists go so far as to say that this does no harm and that if washing and scrubbing fails to shift the blackheads, careful removal by hand is permissible.

Long-term treatment with the tetracyline group of antibiotics is a new and successful form of treatment which works by altering the composition of the sebum so that its level of fatty acids is reduced. Its action in acne is not, therefore, by an antibacterial effect.

As well as frequent washing, the skin needs a lotion which is designed to make it peel and so to open up the blocked pores. The simplest lotion is calamine to which 3 per cent of sulphur has been added; this does not require a doctor's prescription. The calamine and sulphur lotion is put on the skin after the hot wash. When it has dried it is rubbed into the skin so as to increase its peeling effect. Calamine lotion has the added advantage of being a light brown colour which camouflages the spots without giving the appearance of make-up.

Ultra-violet light has a similar action in causing the skin to peel. People with acne should therefore get out in the sun as much as possible. They should also adopt hairstyles which do not screen the sun from the face. A fringe of hair may hide some spots but since it prevents the sun's rays from reaching them they persist. Ultra-violet light can also be obtained from a special lamp, but the time spent under it must be carefully controlled and the eyes must be protected by dark glasses during use.

Sweets and chocolate have often been blamed for making acne worse but diet in any form probably makes very little difference.

In girls, the spots are likely to be worse immediately before the periods, as a result of hormone changes. Stress is another important aggravating factor so that exams may produce an extra crop of spots. Even minor anxieties may make the spots worse, and since in this age group particularly the spots cause severe social embarrassment a vicious circle is set up. This means that for a girl a compromise over cosmetics must be reached; although greasy cosmetics make the spots worse, the use of some cosmetics should be encouraged if this is needed to give her confidence to go out and lead a normal social life.

Sufferers from acne can be helped by knowing that the hormone changes accompanying puberty which produce acne are transitory. When the phase has passed the spots will disappear, though scars caused by deep infection will remain. Merely telling an adolescent that he will grow out of the spots with time and that he must be patient is not enough. By understanding why acne occurs much can be done to keep it down until he has grown out of the liability to these embarrassing spots.

the facts of life 55.

Not so long ago a 'pregnancy doll' was imported into this country. This had a zip front which opened to let out a baby doll lying inside. There was an immediate public outcry, shortly followed by an announcement from the National Union of Small Shopkeepers that the doll had been removed from sale.

Does any of this matter? Possibly. The story suggests that we are going back to the days when adults, because of their own upbringing and embarrassment, refused to talk to children on subjects they found delicate. Pregnancy dolls could be a useful aid in helping parents to explain how the unborn baby grows and develops inside the mother. One is bound to infer that those who reacted against the dolls find pregnancy embarrassing and consider it would not be good for children to know about it.

How very different all this is from the extremely sound advice of Prince Charles when addressing 5,000 businessmen of the Institute of Directors recently. Parents, he said, should be responsible for explaining to their children the complexities of life. 'Do it by reason, logic, persuasion, but don't for God's sake just let children find out by themselves.'

Telling the child means talking about every aspect of life and not only the 'facts' of life. It involves having one's ears tuned to the things he says in order to understand how much he already knows and where his muddles lie. It involves listening before talking and begins as soon as he is able to talk.

Recently, we had a little boy of four in the ward who had had to have several abdominal operations because his bowels were malformed at birth. At this time he had three openings in his abdomen; one was a colostomy for his lower bowel, one was for his upper bowel and the third drained the urine from his bladder. One day, while very seriously ill, he said to a hospital play-specialist: 'I am a girl, I want to sit down and wee-wee.' It would have been easy for someone not trained to listen to children to laugh off the child's remark because of embarrassment. Instead she told the doctors and it gave us all an understanding of the muddle the three holes were creating in the child's mind. Afterwards, working through the play-specialist, it was possible to help him out of his muddle by telling him what it was all about. This was an enormous benefit to the child, who slowly turned the corner. By the end of a year all three openings were closed and he was doing well.

The anxiety created in a child's mind by ignorance is much greater than that produced by learning the truth. It is also much more difficult to tell a child a lie than to tell him the truth. Moreover, a child is almost certain to find out that he has been told a lie and this leaves him uncertain whether, in future, to believe anything that that person tells him.

Some parents try to protect their child from experiencing grief so that if, for example, his pet dies a replacement is immediately bought. This quick action deprives the child of his right to grieve the loss of his pet and may instill in him a belief that the loss of loved ones is not important and that love and loyalty can be quickly shifted.

In some children's wards the death of a child patient is followed by changing all the beds round with the idea that the children won't notice the loss. Nothing could be further from the truth, but it may well prevent the children from asking difficult questions of staff untrained to answer them. The wise ward sister, on this occasion, will spend her day slowly going round the ward sitting on the children's beds and giving them a chance to talk about the death of the child.

The right age to answer a child's questions on any matter is when he first asks about it. If he has not asked questions on important subjects which he is likely to have thought about it is wise to introduce these gently into the conversation in case something has happened to make him feel he can't talk about them.

talking about death 56.

Every child thinks about death, and it will not be long before they start to ask questions about it, exactly as they do about sex. It will be some time before a child understands that death is irreversible, so when a young child tells his mother he wishes she were dead, he will not mean what she thinks; he only wants to get rid of her temporarily.

In the same way that it takes a child many talks to understand about sex, so will it take a long time for him to understand the meaning of death. Accuracy and honesty are essential. If a child's grandmother dies he should not be told that she has gone to sleep. This could lead to fears that he too may disappear when he goes to sleep, or at least to a feeling of guilt that he did not say goodnight to her before she 'went to sleep'.

PARENTAL APPROACHES

The emotions of adults when talking about death are likely to be coloured by fears of the unknown, but a child is much more matter of fact. A young child's reaction to bereavement may seem almost callous by adult standards. A child can easily accept that if everyone went on living the world would soon be so overpopulated that life would be impossible. In other words, death is a necessary part of the cycle of life. He can also understand that some people live longer than others in the same way that some animals live longer than others. Keeping a pet helps a child to be more aware of other lives. Experiencing the loss of a pet can even be a valuable emotional experience, as I have discussed on page 139.

The explanation to a child of what happens after death will depend on the beliefs of the person explaining. A child soon learns that a dead body disintegrates, but whatever a parent's beliefs about life after death may be a child can truthfully be told that the memory and influence of an individual live on for ever. In this sense, death is never the end of the individual.

Studies of children's drawings show that they frequently think of the moment of death as being painful. Their drawings are red from blood and abound in guns and bows and arrows. No doubt this shows an influence of television. A child may be more frightened by anticipating the pain of dying than by the concept of no longer being alive. Children should be told that death is usually painless and that it is the task of doctors and nurses to ensure this when caring for the dying.

The child with a fatal illness needs to have his questions answered honestly. If these are listened to carefully it will frequently be found that he is asking whether he is going to die. If he does ask, he must be given an honest answer, though it may be too painful for his parents to tell him. It sometimes helps if a doctor or nurse does it for them, and then they can go on discussing it with their child afterwards.

People are often shocked that a dying child should ever be told the truth, but he is usually helped by knowing the facts. His parents have been honest with him up till now; why, for the most crucial of all pieces of information, should the truth be withheld? A child can actually help his parents and himself by talking about his impending death and by sharing the feelings which previously they were all experiencing alone.

In western society, where death has become such a taboo subject of conversation, the loss of a child can lead bereaved parents to be shunned by their neighbours, almost as though they have been put in quarantine. Parents need to talk about their lost child, but relatives as well as friends are likely to feel unable to fill this need because of the embarrassment they feel about the subject of death. Such parents need a compassionate friend who will listen to them while they talk about their dead child, for only in this way will they be able to work through their grief. It is this need which has led to the foundation of the Society of the Compassionate Friends, which is composed of bereaved parents who, having worked through their own personal grief, are now able to help others in the same situation.

Parental grief for the dead child can lead to the rejection of his remaining brothers and sisters. Surviving children may thus be exposed to new stresses just when they need all the help their parents can give them in order to work through their own grief.

deprivation 57.

It was not long ago that the term 'deprivation', applied to an individual, referred to the absence or loss of parts or organs. Today, it usually refers to emotional deprivation. Why the change? Is this an indication of a greater understanding by society of the emotional needs of the individual, or is it the result of new pressures?

PARENTAL APPROACHES

Certainly, there is now a greater realization of the emotional stresses which surround us all, but where deprivation is concerned I suspect that the factors causing it are on the increase.

It is probable that most people were made aware of the effects of maternal deprivation by learning of the behaviour of children in hospital when deprived of maternal affection. What is surprising is the time it took for the cause of this behaviour to be understood. How extraordinary that doctors and nurses referred to the silent child in hospital – stunned by separation from mother and home and desperate with feelings of being punished and abandoned, as being a 'good' patient. Small wonder that on returning home the child reacted against his mother, to whom he attributed the blame for being put away. Even now there are parents who, being upset by their child's cries when they leave him in hospital, feel it would be wiser not to visit. Unrestricted visiting – meaning freedom of access at literally any time of day or night – has done much to reduce these problems. But it still needs to be emphasised to parents that the child who cries when they leave is showing a normal reaction, whereas the child who reacts by stunned silence is indicating the depth of his hurt and an urgent need for steps to be taken to remedy the situation. This can be achieved either by his mother sleeping in hospital with him or, if at all possible, by his discharge back home.

All parents should be warned that a child, particularly of the pre-school age, returning home from a stay in hospital may appear 'difficult'. He may react by being aggressive, especially to his mother and to his younger brothers and sisters. He may revert to previous infantile habits such as soiling or wetting and he may refuse to let his mother out of his sight, even insisting that he accompanies her to the lavatory. Small wonder that he no longer trusts her out of his sight in view of what he believes she has done to him.

The child who behaves in this way is reacting

to the loss of a normal maternal relationship. Much more serious is the child who has been deprived of mothering from the start. The ability to mother is something which we learn on our own mother's knee. It is totally different from the technical skills of mothercraft, and far more important.

Individuals learn the art of mothering through their personal experiences of being mothered as children. In the absence of a mother the art can still be learnt through the continued love of a substitute mother. It will not be learnt if the child is cared for by a succession of substitute mothers, as used to happen in orphanages. Such a child is denied the opportunity of experiencing deep maternal affection; consequently, when he becomes an adult his relationships with people are likely to be superficial.

Lack of mothering can occur without the physical loss of a mother. If she is cold and lacking in affection – probably because of her own childhood experiences – she will have a similar damaging effect on her child. This lack is the most catching of influences, being passed on from one generation to the next. It accounts for the majority of parents who batter their children (see below).

Another form of deprivation is play deprivation. The normal baby requires the stimulus of play in order to develop his physical and intellectual powers to the fullest extent. The baby learns through play; a lack of opportunities for play will slow down his learning processes and can prevent his ultimate achievement from realising its maximum potential.

Play does not take place so naturally that a mother automatically plays with her baby. Many mothers in fact need to have the importance of play emphasised, because they have themselves been brought up to think it a waste of time. Play is food for a baby; if he is starved of it when young he may never be able to make up the deficiency.

Whatever the cause of emotional deprivation,

its effect on a child is to create unhappiness and a poor performance.

58. why might I batter my baby?

The idea that a parent might physically assault his or her baby is so repulsive that it is one of the subjects seldom discussed between mothers. Yet it is so common, and the thought of the possibility still commoner, that the majority of mothers have at some time felt like hitting their baby even if they have not actually smacked him. Having once hit him, they feel doubly guilty and yet are very likely to feel too ashamed to tell anyone about it.

It is true that although most mothers have felt like smacking their babies only a minority go on to batter them. Normally, there is an inbuilt mechanism which stops the mother at the last moment, however much her child is infuriating her; she goes and makes herself a cup of tea instead.

The reason why this minority of mothers batter their babies has been established. Almost all had an unhappy childhood – they were not mothered. Mothering is learnt on your mother's knee and by her whole approach to you as a young child. The girl or boy who was denied this experience does not know how to mother (or father) her own child. Such a mother will have false expectations of her child. She may expect her baby automatically to make her happy – to give her something which was denied to her as a baby. She may hate her baby because he represents herself as a baby and this was a very unhappy time of her life.

She will demand a loving response from him. When he cries she will feel that he is accusing her of not knowing how to make him happy. This will cause her to be angry with him so that she is determined to make the baby stop crying, even if it is the last thing she does to him; tragically, it occasionally is.

Battering is something which happens in all

classes of people; it is not confined to the working classes. The reason why it occurs more often in this class is that overcrowding and therefore exasperation is likely to be greater. Moreover, if a mother who is well off feels like battering her baby she can take evasive action and have a nanny or at least a baby sitter.

For some mothers, the results of these problems are not that they physically batter their babies but that they are unable to love them. Consequently, the baby fails to thrive. Babies who are not handled lovingly lose their interest in life and go off their feeds. They seldom smile but stare passively around. This is emotional battering, and in the long run it may be even more traumatic for the child than physical battering.

The prevention of battering lies in the provision of a normal happy childhood – the best preparation for normal parenthood. For those who were denied this, much can still be done to help once the mechanism for their feelings is understood. A knowledge of normal psychology helps. Many mothers are frightened by being left alone with their babies and need to talk out these fears. Many mothers feel guilty that they do not love their babies totally the moment they are born. They have been brought up on the myth of instant love – which seldom happens. Love at first sight applies to some babies as it does for some future husbands, but mostly it takes time to fall in love.

Further help involves the provision of mothering for the mother who is liable to batter her baby. This mothering could be provided by an understanding mother-in-law, but more often it needs to come from an outsider. Husbands can help by understanding the problem but they are unlikely to change to the extent of providing support for wives who to date have not received this.

This outsider has been called a 'mothering aide'. She does not have to be specially trained but she does need to be someone with a loving nature who has already had experience of successfully bringing up a family. She has to be ready to absorb the demands put on her by the mother at risk and to be available to help at any time of day or night as well as by making frequent visits on her own. She must not pick up the crying baby from his mother's arms since if she stopped the baby crying by this action she would confirm still more strongly the mother's feelings of her own inadequacy.

A mothering aide cannot possibly care for more than one mother at a time and even this will put such a strain on her that she must be able to talk out the problems in a group of other mothering aides, led by a doctor or social worker.

People who work as mothering aides should be paid for what they do. How suitable that a successful grandmother should put her greatest skills into practice again to help in this way.

The important thing with mothers at risk of battering is that they should be recognised early, perhaps even before they are aware of their own feelings. The question 'does your baby make you angry?' is answered by the normal mother that it only makes her want to cuddle him more. The mother who might batter her baby is likely, when asked directly, to be aware that her baby does make her feel angry.

The baby who cries all day has not got 'wind' and is unlikely to be hungry since feeding is the first thing his mother will have tried. Almost certainly his crying is a reflection of her turmoil which, if unrecognised, can lead to battering.

Much can be done to help, both by prevention and by treatment where the problem has already occurred. Such mothers need help, not punishment. Society has yet to learn – and must be educated – about this subject.

59. children who wake at night

From the number of letters I get on this subject, it is clear that it is still one of the major anxieties for parents. The first need, in order to get the problem into perspective, is to clear the air of a number of old-fashioned ideas which still pervade the subject of children and their sleep.

Children do not need sleep in order to grow. There is no truth in the statement that you only grow when you are asleep. Growth goes on throughout the day and night. Then there is the remark that a child's brain will tire if he doesn't sleep. This is another bit of nonsense. A child will sleep when he needs to, and more or less despite anything you can do to stop him. It is the anxious and depressed adult who suffers from insomnia, not the child. The only time an adult might stop a child from sleeping is when he has so over-emphasised the need for sleep that the child worries because he cannot get off to sleep. Once such a child is given a bedside reading lamp and is told he can read for as long as he wants, he will go off to sleep without difficulty– though he may leave the light on!

Another fallacious idea is that there is a fixed amount of sleep required by a child and that the younger he is the more hours of sleep he needs. Many parents need far more sleep than their children and it is perfectly all right for them to go to bed first.

When it comes down to basic facts, the only real reason why parents should want their children to sleep is to give themselves a rest. This is a very normal and human reason which, once accepted, reduces the problem of the child waking at night. If parents can get their rest without the child actually being asleep this is just as good. This requires a much less rigid approach to bedtime since if, for example, a child is happily reading a book he can be left to do so or told he can read in bed – not that he must go to sleep.

Staying up to watch television always raises strong parental feelings, but in itself it is not a bad thing provided the activity can be kept in perspective. First, it must be agreed that in the evening parents choose whether or not the television is on and that they select the programme. This could result in the child watching an educative programme which he would otherwise have missed.

One of the fears is that if a child stays up late at night he will be too tired to get up for school in the morning. This may well be true, but I think it is more often bound up with school than with the hours of sleep. I so often meet children whose parents are lenient about later hours of going to bed during the holidays and I am told that in the holidays the child is up with the lark. Surely it is common to all of us that when we have something exciting to do we have little difficulty in getting out of bed?

This leads us to the baby, usually of toddler age, who wakes in the early hours of the morning wanting to play. He has had enough sleep and he starts to do just what he enjoys most – play. This is not harmful; in fact from the baby's point of view it is a positive advantage. Since he learns through play he is volunteering to do extra 'homework'.

Of course, this is a nuisance for his parents whose sleep is disturbed. The disturbance can be lessened if the child has a room of his own and if he has toys put near him which may occupy him for a time when he first wakes, particularly if these are not of the squeaky variety. Putting such a child to bed as late as is practical may lessen the problem, but in the end there are some toddlers who are so demanding that one or other parent has to go and play with them. Fortunately, this task can be shared so that each parent is not up every night. It helps, too, to know that this period will not go on for ever: usually it only lasts a matter of months. Most encouraging of all is the fact that it is bright children who behave in this way – the dull ones are much more likely to sleep through the night because they have not got the same amount of natural curiosity – the talent that excites the bright ones into greater activity.

I am quite clear that if I was buying a baby I would choose one who woke up to play in the middle of the night!

Finally, there is the baby who in the early months of life wakes in the night. At this age the baby cries out since he is too young to play on his own. The first thing is to go to him. Never leave a baby crying because of the idea that you will spoil him if you pick him up. He is crying for some very good reason and he needs immediate comfort.

If he can sleep in a room of his own, his parents will get more sleep because his mother, particularly, will not be able to hear his first snufflings as he begins to wake which would immediately alert her and cut down her own amount of sleep if they shared the same room.

The young baby who wakes very probably needs a feed. I am always surprised by the number of babies who drop their night feed quite early, considering that their digestion is not adjusted differently for day and night. To begin with it is a matter of trying out a number of tricks to see which works best with your baby. You can try going to bed early and not waking him for his 10 p.m. feed and see if this gives you more sleep than if you stay up until you have given him a feed at 10 o'clock. It is all a matter of trial and error, accepting that this is a running-in period and that the more placid a mother is over the whole of her baby's management, the less he is likely to cry.

forcing a child to stay away 60.

'Miranda is ten in September, a highly intelligent, quite precocious child who during the last year or so has rigidly refused to stay away the night with friends – however well she knows them and however near they are to us. Should we force her? She does enjoy herself before going to bed and on awakening. But she cries at the thought of going, has to be forced and then says she has a tummy ache when she goes to bed.

PARENTAL APPROACHES

'She cannot explain why she does not like going. We ask her whether she thinks we are going to disappear. "No", she says. But she does admit that she is terrified that the others in the house will go to sleep before her. A year ago I did force her to go to Scotland for ten days to stay with her godmother whom she knows very well. She flew there and almost had to come back the next day. There was an awful scene but in the end she stayed and enjoyed herself but she does not want to go again and we are not forcing her.

'Twice recently I have made her go away locally but each time she has telephoned at 9.30 asking me to collect her. Once I refused and the child's father was very cross with her; she stayed but said "it was like being in prison".

'I do feel she is being childish but she does get so upset. And she misses out on so many opportunities of staying with friends and relations which I think is a pity. Should we hope she will grow out of it?

'By the way, she plans to go to Norway after Christmas with the au pair for two weeks, but she wants this as she says the au pair babysits for her and that is quite a different matter from staying with friends down the road.'

This letter illustrates how easy it is for a mother to try to force her child to do something against the child's wishes in the belief that it is 'good' for the child. The clue to Miranda's problem is that she is frightened of going to sleep unless she is with someone she knows very well. She bears out her mother's description that she is highly intelligent since she had been able to put some of her fears into words: she is frightened that everyone in the house will go to sleep before her.

It would be the worst thing possible for her to be forced to go away against her wishes – she will certainly not grow out of it that way. Miranda will gain confidence by going away with people she loves and trusts. It is a great compliment to the au pair girl that Miranda has made plans to go with her to Norway. This should persuade her mother that it is not the surroundings which matter but that Miranda needs to be with people with whom she feels safe. Nor is it distance, since she feels safer in Norway than in a house down the road. Miranda has expressed all this very vividly in saying that the au pair girl babysits for her. For all her precocity Miranda has babyish fears and it is no use telling her not to be a baby. You might as well tell her to be British and brave.

Children can be helped through their fears by exactly the opposite approach from the 'stand up and be brave' concept. By subtlety it is possible to make the fear smaller and, therefore, the child bigger. If a child is frightened of the dark he can be given a night-light and have the door of his room left open. In this way the dark becomes less fearful and the whole approach more positive in its help for the child.

Miranda is only nine years old and yet her mother describes her as being 'childish'. Surely she has every reason to be! How harsh that the father of the child with whom Miranda stayed once should fall into the same trap and become very cross when she telephoned her mother to ask if she could come home. Has he never been frightened, and if so has he been helped by people getting angry with him for his fears? Small wonder that Miranda felt imprisoned when her mother's friend treated her in this way.

Miranda's tummyache is also instructive. If she is forced into going away she says she has tummyache when she goes to bed. Why did her mother use the phrase 'says she has tummyache' instead of writing that she had a tummyache. One wonders if she believes Miranda has made it up, but that is certainly not the case. Stomachs are an accurate barometer for feelings; many vivid descriptions such as 'butterflies in the stomach' bear this out. If Miranda had fabricated her pain she would be a malingerer but her story does not suggest that.

The probable explanation for tummyaches associated with anxiety is that the waves of bowel movement driving the food through the intestine have been increased in force, and reach the level of consciousness so that they can be felt. This is borne out by the association of diarrhoea with anxiety. The basement of the examination hall used by medical students for their exams is full of lavatories.

Miranda's mother should direct her efforts towards finding out what happened to Miranda a year ago to make her frightened of going away (if indeed this is a new occurrence). She should also ask herself why she feels so strongly that Miranda should stay away. She can, however, be assured that Miranda's behaviour is quite normal and that no good will result from a rigid or unsympathetic attitude over Miranda's present fears.

61. thinking about holidays

The first necessity where holidays are concerned is for parents to work out their own wishes and then see how these are likely to fit in with those of their children. If you know that leaving your baby in the care of someone else while you are on holiday will make you very unhappy, then take him with you. On the other hand, if you are longing for a rest from your child or children and have made adequate arrangements for their care while you are away – possibly best of all with one of their grandparents – then there is no reason why you should not go off on your own.

There is really nowhere in the world that is unsafe for a baby. Don't be put off by the idea that he won't be able to stand the heat – he will easily be able to tolerate anything you can, provided you dress him appropriately and don't leave him in the burning sun before he is able to move himself away from it when he wants.

Similarly, babies can travel in any variety of transport so this need not influence your decision. When going out to dinner with friends, my wife, seated on the pillion seat of my motorbike, used to tow the pram containing our first child – not that I would recommend this mode of transport, but we were always much happier if he came with us.

After the baby stage it would be natural for you always to have your children with you on holiday. The problem then becomes one of where to stay. Possibly the least traumatic for all concerned is camping or caravanning. I must admit that I prefer the luxury of a caravan and feel it is the ideal way of enjoying a holiday with very young children. When travelling long distances on the Continent it makes the break for a mid-day meal such a luxury. We always used to hire a caravan and for many years my children would proudly and correctly state that they knew Paris better than London. The Bois de Bologne has a splendid camping site and there was never any difficulty in getting the occupants of a neighbouring caravan to keep an eye on the sleeping children while my wife and I went out in the evening.

If you are able to afford it you could rent a villa instead of a caravan, but I would avoid a hotel unless your young children are perfect. Living in a tent, caravan or villa means that you can look after your children in your normal way. If you are in a hotel you are going to be influenced by the reproving glances of other hotel guests and you will find yourself trying to make your children behave at meals with a strictness which never existed at home. You cannot expect your child suddenly to have perfect table manners, to eat strange food and not to play about while waiting between courses.

The father of the family will probably have to sort himself out a bit while on holiday with the children; the chances are that he will never have had them around him for so long at a stretch before. The different code of rules he demands for the children's behaviour may show up more obviously when he is around all day and will need working out with his wife before the children get into a muddle. He may feel guilty when he realises how much his wife has to cope with every day, though this may still not stop him from going off fishing on his own in order to get some peace.

Sharing a holiday with another family is often a success provided you know beforehand that both the adults and the children get on well. This arrangement means that you can share the baby-sitting so that one couple is always free in the evening. It also means that if the men are bored and want to go off together there are two wives to keep each other company.

Going to the seaside is not automatically a pleasure for children. The toddler may be very frightened of the sea, especially when he sees you disappearing into this strange thing. While an older child enjoys the freedom of the sea and sands a toddler may be frightened, cold and itching from the sand in his pants. You have to work for your children's enjoyment at the sea-side just as you do everywhere else, and you have to guard them even more carefully.

If you do decide that you want to leave your young children in the care of someone else while you go away, but are worried by the possible effect it may have on them, there are several points to consider. You may wonder whether their subconscious fear and anger caused by your temporary loss will mean they reject you on your return; they might even seem not to recognise you. Alternatively, they could become so insecure that it later becomes impossible to leave them with a babysitter again as it causes them so much distress.

The way to reduce the likelihood of any of these repercussions is to make sure you arrange for them to be looked after by one person, who must be motherly and understanding. This may be a grandmother, but could equally well be the right sort of person from an agency. Whoever looks after them, it should be one person only all time you are away, and if possible she and the children should get to know each other before you go. It is much better for the children to be looked after in their own home, where they are surrounded by familiar things, than for them to be sent away to a strange house.

What about holidays for older children away from their parents – either alone with friends or in a group such as a Scout or Guide camp? The usual rules must apply: only send your child if he really wants to go. On no account send him alone to toughen him up or to try to hasten the speed with which he becomes independent. If you send him against his will he will feel he is being pushed out; his developing independence will only be delayed by the experience.

health on holiday 62.

If you are going abroad for your holiday there will be preparations to make. From a health point of view this involves extra immunisation. This takes time because of the need for intervals between doses, so you should start several weeks before your holiday. Immunisation requirements are complicated but have been made easier by an excellent leaflet issued for travellers by the Department of Health. This should be supplied to you by your travel agent or it is available on direct application to the Department of Health at the Elephant and Castle, London, SE1. There are only three diseases for which compulsory vaccination is required: smallpox, yellow fever and cholera. Whether or not any or all of these are required depends on the countries you are visiting.

In addition, if you are going outside Europe, other than to Canada and the USA, you should be vaccinated against poliomyelitis. This disease attacks adults just as much as children and is common in developing countries. Tragedies have occurred when unvaccinated travellers have caught poliomyelitis.

Vaccination against typhoid (TAB) is a wise precaution if you are going to a country where the water supply and the standard of hygiene are less advanced than they are in Britain. It should be the rule for travellers to developing countries, and should be considered if you are going to one of the Mediterranean countries or to eastern Europe. Modern techniques of giving TAB cause much less pain than that endured by the troops in the last war, who received an injection into the muscle.

Malaria still exists in some countries outside Europe, so you should enquire about this in relation to your journey. If you are visiting or passing through an area where malaria occurs you should take anti-malaria drugs.

Although tetanus is rare, it is wise to have a shot every five years so as to keep up the protection, especially if you are likely to go to a developing country.

Having arrived at your holiday resort, and assuming you are lucky enough to have good weather, sunburn is the next problem. The risks are lessened if you have been able to acclimatise your children in the sun at home, but this still won't prevent the effects of the Mediterranean sun. Half an hour in the sun is enough for the first two or three days and even this may be too long for those with fair skin. The difficulty in persuading children of the risks of sunburn is that it does not hurt until some hours after exposure to the sun, though it may help if you can point out someone on the beach who is obviously suffering from it.

Sun creams provide a certain amount of protection and should certainly be used but they must not be relied on to give complete protection. There is no alternative to playing in the shade or, if a child is exposed to the sun, to wearing a light shirt with his bathing suit. This should be kept on when he is in the water, since the reflection of the sun's rays off the surface of the water may even increase the risk when in the water.

Take some calamine lotion with you on holiday since this is the most useful and soothing first aid remedy for anyone who does get burnt. Aspirin may be needed to relieve the pain.

Stomach upsets are the next problem, producing 'traveller's diarrhoea'. These are due either to a change of diet or to actual germs in the food or water. Probably the change to a larger, richer and more spicy diet is the more common cause. Fortunately, this usually clears up in about two days and although it is a nuisance the victim doesn't feel ill. Plenty of fluid to replace what is lost in the stools, and a light diet if the person feels like it, is all that is necessary. Antibiotics make no difference but a chalk mixture (Kaolin) may make the motions solid more quickly.

It is quite a different matter if the person who catches diarrhoea feels ill with it. In this case it may be due to one of the varieties of dysentery. Medical help is needed to identify the cause and to provide the right treatment. Since medical treatment outside Britain can be very expensive it is wise to take out medical insurance before leaving for the holiday.

One last important point to remember is that if you fall ill shortly after you return from a holiday abroad you must be sure to tell your doctor where you have been, as you may have picked up an unusual infection. This is particularly important in relation to malaria.

keeping the peace on the road 63.

It depends to some extent on the temperament of the adults, particularly the driver, whether motoring with children is regarded as a nightmare or a pleasure. But however placid the driver, the safety of everyone in the car and of fellow road-users requires steps to be taken to ensure as peaceful a car load as is practical.

Children should never travel in the front of a car. Adult seat belts do not fit a child; worst of all is the child on someone's lap who would so easily be thrown forward into the windscreen by a sudden stop, let alone an accident. If a child must sit on someone's lap, be sure that this is in the back seat.

The right thing is to provide special safety belts in the back for the older children and safety seats attached to the back seat for older babies and toddlers. Young babies can travel in their carry-cots, but these must be safely wedged so that they cannot slide forward. In a four-door car the rear doors must be fitted with safety catches so that they can only be opened from the outside.

To increase their safety, the children should be entertained if not asleep. Sleeping children are best for peace, and it is sometimes worth planning a night journey to achieve this.

Entertainment has to be planned in advance, the type of activity depending on the age and interests of the children concerned. Each child will need his own flat surface on which to play some of his games. The ideal is a deep-sided tray. A pad and pencil, books and comics, jig-saws, puzzles, threading beads and hand puppets all help. Something new, even if this is only a notebook, often keeps a child occupied for longer than something familiar.

Older children can have their interest held by becoming involved in the journey itself. Competitions involving car numbers or different makes of car mean that each oncoming car has especial interest. Road signs and inn signs can all be brought into competitions. I Spy books make use of all these. Some children will be absorbed for a time by following the route on the map, especially if they are given the responsibility for directing the driver. A car compass will add to the interest.

It is a good idea for each child to have his own bag in which to keep his possessions while travelling. This should lead to fewer quarrels over ownership. Cleaning up the debris at intervals reduces the clutter which otherwise makes play more difficult and increases the likelihood of arguments.

How frequently you break the journey depends on the driver's temperament and the children's behaviour. The important thing is to choose a spot where the children can have a real run around so that they let off steam. Stopping in a lay-by or on the edge of a busy road provides little change of scenery and demands another exhausting watch for their safety.

Picnic meals are usually more fun and more relaxing than long waits in stuffy restaurants. Snacks between meals will help to ward off boredom but choose foods which are not too filling, such as crisps, salty biscuits, cheese in little packets and apples. Chewing gum and sweets which last a long time should also help. Be sure to bring plenty to drink since children seem to get particularly thirsty on journeys.

For bottlefed babies the simplest and safest method is to use pre-packed feeds in disposable bottles. It does not matter if this is not his usual feed – babies can tolerate any make of feed – but it would be as well to try him out on it beforehand to make sure he does not make life more difficult by refusing it altogether.

When using your own mixed feed, it is best to make this up beforehand, keeping it cold in an insulated container and pouring it into a clean bottle just before use. It is unsafe to keep the milk warm for several hours since this gives any germs present the chance to multiply. The milk can be given cold to the baby – few babies refuse a feed because it is cold. It is an adult concept that a baby's bottle must contain milk that is warm.

Washing and changing a baby while travelling can be a problem. However, disposable napkins and tissues make a world of difference. Topping and tailing is all that is required and pre-packed damp cloths can replace soap and water for cleaning. A big plastic bag for all the soiled articles will make life easier. For the child who is pot-trained a new pot has been especially designed for use when travelling. It incorporates a disposable plastic bag which solves the difficult problem of emptying.

Travel sickness is much more of a problem with children than with adults, which means you can anticipate improvements as they get older. Give the child a light meal before starting and try to let him have it an hour before the journey begins. There should not be an embargo on food while travelling but dry biscuits, glucose sweets and similar snacks are best if food is wanted.

Reading increases the likelihood of travel sickness, but games which involve looking out of the car and concentration should help. An atmosphere of calm, as opposed to one of fear that the child will be sick, is essential. You will need to be armed with a big plastic bag in case he is sick but this should be kept out of the way since its mere sight may induce vomiting in a susceptible child. The most effective pill to prevent travel sickness is one containing hyoscine, which should be given half an hour before the start of the journey.

Excitement increases the liability to travel sickness. Some children are only sick when travelling to their holiday home and not on the return journeys presumably because they are less excited.

A car journey is an opportunity to teach a child general points about safety on the road. Let him first sit in the driver's seat when the car is stationary so that he can learn something about blind spots where the driver could not see a child. This will help him appreciate the dangers of playing near parked cars which might reverse and injure him because he was invisible to the driver. During the car journey he can learn that a car cannot stop instantly so that he appreciates the dangers of suddenly stepping into the road in front of a car. During the journey there are likely to be several opportunities to point out the safe or the dangerous behaviour of children on the road.